T0315406

REHABILITATION OF VISUAL DISORDERS AFTER BRAIN INJURY

Rehabilitation of Visual Disorders after Brain Injury

Josef Zihl

*Institute of Psychology, Neuropsychology, Ludwig-
Maximilians University, Munich, Germany
and
Max-Planck Institute of Psychiatry, Munich, Germany*

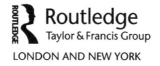

Routledge
Taylor & Francis Group
LONDON AND NEW YORK

First published 2000 by Psychology Press Ltd.

Published 2021 by Routlege
2 Park Square, Milton Park, Abingdon, Oxon OX14 4RN
605 Third Avenue, New York, NY 10017

Routledge is an imprint of the Taylor & Francis Group, an informa business

British Library Cataloguing in Publication Data

A catalogue record for this book is available from the British Library

Typeset by Graphicraft Limited, Hong Kong

ISBN 13: 978-0-86377-898-8 (hbk)
ISBN 13: 978-0-86377-899-5 (pbk)
ISSN 1466-6340 (Neuropsychological Rehabilitation: A Modular Handbook)

Contents

Series preface

Rehabilitation is a process whereby people, who have been injured by injury or illness, work together with health service staff and others to achieve their optimum level of physical, psychological, social and vocational well-being (McLellan, 1991). It includes all measures aimed at reducing the impact of handicapping and disabling conditions and at enabling disabled people to return to their most appropriate environment (WHO, 1986; Wilson, 1997). It also includes attempts to alter impairment in underlying cognitive and brain systems by the provision of systematic, planned experience to the damaged brain (Robertson & Murre, in press). The above views apply also to neuropsychological rehabilitation, which is concerned with the assessment, treatment and natural recovery of people who have sustained an insult to the brain.

Neuropsychological rehabilitation is influenced by a number of fields both from within and without psychology. Neuropsychology, behavioural psychology and cognitive psychology have each played important roles in the development of current rehabilitation practice. So too have findings from studies of neuroplasticity, linguistics, geriatric medicine, neurology and other fields. Our discipline, therefore, is not confined to one conceptual framework; rather, it has a broad theoretical base.

We hope that this broad base is reflected in the modular handbook. The first book was by Roger Barker and Stephen Dunnett which set the scene by talking about 'Neural repair, transplantation and rehabilitation'. This second title, by Josef Zihl, addresses visual disorders after brain injury. Forthcoming titles include volumes on specific cognitive functions such as language, memory and motor skills, together with social and personality aspects of neuropsychological rehabilitation and behavioural approaches to rehabilitation. Other titles will follow as this is the kind of handbook at can be added to over the years.

Although each volume will be based on a strong theoretical foundation relevant to the topic in question, the main thrust of a majority of the books will be the development of practical, clinical methods of rehabilitation arising out of this research enterprise.

The series is aimed at neuropsychologists, clinical psychologists and other rehabilitation specialists such as occupational therapists, speech and language pathologists, rehabilitation physicians and other disciplines involved in the rehabilitation of people with brain injury.

Neuropsychological rehabilitation is at an exciting stage in its development. On the one hand, we have a huge growth of interest in functional imaging techniques to tell us about the basic processes going on in the brain. On the other hand, the past few years have seen the introduction of a number of theoretically driven approaches to cognitive rehabilitation from the fields of language, memory, attention and perception. In addition to both the above, there is a growing recognition from health services that rehabilitation is an integral part of a health care system. Of course, alongside the recognition of the need for rehabilitation is the view that any system has to be evaluated. To those of us working with brain injured people including those with dementia, there is a feeling that things are moving forward. This series, we hope, is one reflection of this move and the integration of theory and practice.

REFERENCES

McLellan, D.L. (1991). Functional recovery and the principles of disability medicine. In M. Swash & J. Oxbury (Eds), *Clinical neurology*. Edinburgh: Churchill Livingstone.

Robertson, I.H., & Murre, J.M.J. (in press). Rehabilitation of brain damage: Brain plasticity and principles of guided recovery. *Psychological Bulletin*.

Wilson, B.A. (1997). Cognitive rehabilitation: How it is and how it might be. *Journal of the International Neuropsychological Society*, 3, 487–496.

World Health Organisation (1986). Optimum care of disabled people. *Report of a WHO meeting*, Turku, Finland.

BARBARA A. WILSON
IAN H. ROBERTSON

Preface

When one writes a book, one is often full of enthusiasm at the beginning, but disillusioned at the end. As soon as the first draft is finished, one wonders whether one has achieved one's objectives—at least to a certain extent—each time one reads the manuscript to revise and improve it. Statements may turn more and more into suppositions, conclusions may lose their strictness and general significance, and in the end only few results may survive as clear, unequivocal facts. It is nevertheless a great adventure to write a book on a topic to which one has dedicated so many years of research and practical work. In addition to my research into the effects of focal brain injuries on visual capacities, I have also always been interested to find out whether or not the visual deficits caused by brain injuries are irreversible. The study of processes of recovery and substitution of function can offer exciting insights into the brain's plasticity, i.e. its potential for functional reorganisation. Since visual perception has always been my favourite research subject, it seemed reasonable to concentrate on the recovery and substitution of this modality. I started working on the research reported in this monograph more or less 20 years ago. It is not surprising that it mostly focuses on patients with visual field disorders as these patients represent by far the largest group. Therefore, it was possible to study treatment effects in quite a large number of patients and to further improve the procedures of treatment (I personally prefer the terms "training" and "systematic practice"). Other visual disorders are not very common; the observations reported have the character of single case studies. However, is it not a common clinical experience that a patient with an uncommon disorder is referred to the "specialist", who is not only expected to identify the exact kind of disorder, but also to know how to treat it? Even though one cannot always fall back on existing cases, it is a great challenge for a clinical neuroscientist to try what appears almost impossible. Of course, observations in single patients cannot be generalised in the same way as studies including larger groups of patients. However, it is quite legitimate to draw the tentative conclusion that even patients with uncommon visual disorders, such as Balint's syndrome or visual agnosia, may also benefit from systematic practice. (Visual neglect has not been considered in this monograph because a special volume shall be dedicated to this syndrome and its treatment. For the management of visual hallucinations after brain injury see Zihl & Kennard, 1986.) The scientist's interest in a patient's functional disorder and the professional's responsibility accurately to assess and effectively treat the patient hopefully enable us to develop appropriate methods for rehabilitation or to improve already existing procedures. There should be no therapeutic nihilism in neuropsychological rehabilitation. I would be more than happy if the experiences and observations reported in this monograph supported other colleagues' work in the field and stimulated further developments.

I am greatly indebted to all the patients participating in the various studies for their trust, motivation and patience. I acknowledge with gratitude the food for thought many colleagues gave me in discussing critical issues (and in rehabilitation research, there are so many critical issues!). I am also indebted to Mrs. Christel Schmid who assisted with assessing and training the patients, as well as with recording and analysing the eye movements and preparing the corresponding figures. I would also like to thank Mrs. Anne Wendl for preparing all the other figures. I am grateful for the continued support of the Max-Planck Institute of Psychiatry and the Deutsche Forschungsgemeinschaft. Part of the work has been supported by SFB 462. Last but not least, I appreciate the care that Psychology Press has taken in publishing this monograph.

CHAPTER ONE

Introduction

From the very beginning of neuroscience, vision research has mainly been concerned with the elucidation of the nature of various visual deficits and the identification of the location of brain injury responsible for these deficits (for a comprehensive review, see Grüsser & Landis, 1991). Early clinical reports on patients showing selective visual loss following posterior brain injury have suggested that visual functions are cortically distributed, a concept that many years later has been verified on the basis of combined anatomical, electrophysiological, and behavioural evidence (Desimone & Ungerleider, 1989; Felleman & van Essen, 1991; Zeki, 1978, 1993). Enormous progress has been made in understanding the neurobiological basis of visual perception, and it is meanwhile generally accepted that the visual cortex is functionally specialised and builds up flexible networks to subserve complex visual abilities, such as recognising objects or orienting in space (Corbetta, Miezin, Shulman, & Petersen, 1993; Tootell, Dale, Sereno, & Malach, 1996). The neuropsychology of vision is still a major topic in neuroscience, and the questions of how the different lower and higher level "processing units" integrate pieces of information, how they co-operate by various interactions to achieve and maintain coherence of visual perception in time and space, and how they are influenced by attention and intention etc., are exciting and very promising research topics for the next few years (see Cowey, 1994, and Driver & Mattingley, 1995, for reviews).

In contrast to the numerous contributions to the understanding of cerebral organisation of visual perception, few, however, are devoted to the study of recovery of visual function in patients with acquired brain injury. This, at first sight, is difficult to understand given the fact that, for example, between 20% and 40% of patients with stroke suffer from visual disorders (Hier, Mondlock, &

Caplan, 1983a; Sarno & Sarno, 1979). Furthermore, visual disorders may affect cognitive performance (Uzzell, Dolinskas, & Langfitt, 1988) and may reduce the effect of rehabilitation measures, thereby impairing vocational rehabilitation (Groswasser, Cohen, & Blankstein, 1990; Reding & Potes, 1988). The reason for this is certainly not the missing interest in the recovery of vision and visual rehabilitation, and furthermore cannot be due to a lack of acknowledgement of this field of brain research. As early as 1867, Zagorski reported the case of a 35-year-old lady who complained of loss of vision on the left side. Perimetric testing revealed a complete left-sided hemianopia, probably caused by a right-sided occipital haemorrhage. Eight days later the patient noticed return of light vision in the left hemifield; 6 weeks later she reported to have full vision again. Perimetric testing of visual fields was performed in intervals of about 1 week. The results were in agreement with the report given by the patient: The region of blindness shrank successively and vision eventually returned to the left hemifield (see Fig. 1.1). This is probably the first report on recovery of vision after brain injury. In their *Handbook for neurologists and ophthalmologists* Wilbrand and Saenger (1917) dedicated a comprehensive chapter to the incidence and course of homonymous hemianopia. According to their observations, in patients with complete cortical blindness, vision recovered first in one hemifield; a few cases later showed complete return of vision. In most of the cases, recovery of vision took place within hours or days; in some patients, however, the process of recovery was much slower and was not completed for several weeks. A similar course was observed in cases with homonymous hemianopia. In the same year (1917), Poppelreuter (1917/1990) published his monograph on visual disturbances after occipital gunshot wounds, in which he not only reported the results of his detailed testing of visual disorders, but also his observations on spontaneous recovery and on the effect of systematic treatment. Poppelreuter's approach was experimentally oriented and at the same time was a very pragmatic one. This is exemplified by his statement (p. 5) that "any intervention should, at the very least, have as its aim that the man should again be able to converse comprehensibly, to write his own letters, to read a newspaper, and to calculate his expenses by himself". Poppelreuter pointed out that functional impairments in the acute stage may often be exaggerated. However, complete spontaneous recovery was the exception rather than the rule; rehabilitation measures were therefore required in most of his patients. Poppelreuter was aware of the difficulty of attributing an improvement unequivocally to the treatment (p. 240): "Only exact control of the effect [of treatment] offers a substantial argument for the systematic training effect over a short period of time, namely using a work task which remains constant." He developed training methods especially aimed at improving reading in patients with visual field loss. He had noticed that parafoveal field loss not only impaired the perception of words but also the guidance of reading eye movements. Therefore he taught patients to compensate for their field loss by systematically shifting fixation from the beginning to the

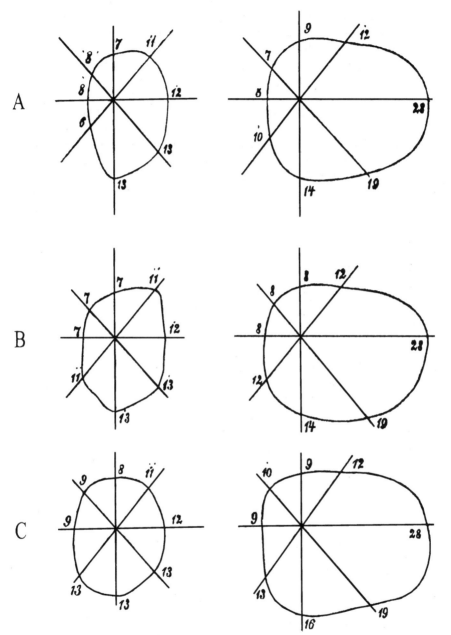

FIG. 1.1 Spontaneous recovery of the left hemifield in Zagorski's case (1867). Left panel: Visual field of left eye, right panel: visual field of the right eye. A: Outcome of perimetric testing on 11 June 1867; B: on 26 June 1867; C: on 5 July 1867. On 27 July, Zagorksi found complete recovery of vision in the left hemifield.

3

end of a line. The resulting improvement in reading is the first known example for the substitution of cerebral visual loss by oculomotor activities. According to Poppelreuter, the substitution of one function (the parafoveal visual field) by another (eye movement) is crucially dependent on whether, under normal circumstances, the substituting function also contributes to the performance in question.

Poppelreuter's observations on the recovery of vision after brain injury and his experiences with the systematic treatment of visually disabled, brain-injured patients were for the most part neglected in the literature, as was the aspect of recovery of visual function in patients with occipital injury. Even in the classic monograph by Teuber, Battersby, and Bender (1960) on visual disturbances in a similar group of cases, namely World War II soldiers with missile wounds to the brain, only few qualitative data are reported on the recovery of visual functions, and no attempts were made to treat the patients. In a later article, Teuber (1975) reported follow-up observations in 520 cases with known brain injuries incurred in World War II or in Korea or Vietnam. He confirmed Poppelreuter's observation that vision can reappear in affected visual field regions.

In contrast to the diminishing interest in the study of recovery of vision after brain injury in man, there was growing interest among brain researchers on the effect of experimental lesions to brain structures subserving vision in animals. It was especially Klüver (1942) who studied the effect of experimentally induced localised lesions on vision in monkeys and found that bilateral occipital injury results in a profound but not total loss of processing of visual information. A "sufficiently long period of training" was, however, required before the monkey was able, for example, to locate objects in space. A famous single case study on a rhesus monkey, Helen, from whom the striate cortex was almost totally removed bilaterally, and who was studied intensively over a period of 8 years (Humphrey, 1974) revealed that the monkey could regain an effective, though limited, degree of visually guided behaviour by practice in her natural environments. Cowey (1967) and Weiskrantz and Cowey (1970) showed convincingly that practice can reduce the size of a cortical, but not a retinal, scotoma in monkeys, as defined by the animal's ability to detect light targets. An even more complete and specific recovery of vision could be demonstrated by Mohler and Wurtz (1977). Deficits in detecting flashes in the cortical scotoma region and in the accuracy of saccadic eye movements directed towards them, disappeared 6 weeks after the lesions were performed. Again, systematic practice was necessary for recovery, which was mainly observed in the portion of the scotoma that had been subjected to practice. Thus, occipital lesions need not always result in an irreversible loss of vision, but systematic treatment is required for its return. Of course, the results obtained in animal studies cannot directly be transferred to patients. It has, for example, been shown that patients can also accurately respond to light stimuli presented in their cortical scotoma. For the demonstration of this phenomenon which has been coined "blindsight", because patients are never aware of the presence of the target, special testing conditions are required, and typically patients show this capacity only after systematic practice (for a review, see Weiskrantz, 1986). It is still an open issue whether this "residual visual capacity" is due to recovery, represents residual functioning of spared visual cortex, or represents a visual function that is subserved by extrageniculo-striate mechanisms that were not affected by injury. However, "blindsight" does not seem to reduce patients' visual disability because they cannot make use of this sub- or unconscious visual function (Zihl, 1980). Therefore, although there is no doubt that in these cases, like in monkeys with cortical scotoma, visual processing takes place in the "blind" field region, nobody would go so far as to consider a patient showing blindsight "visually rehabilitated". Likewise, the methods of practice used to uncover this type of visual processing cannot be considered appropriate for the treatment of patients with visual field loss due to occipital brain injury. Nevertheless, brain lesion research in primates has contributed substantially to the understanding of the recovery of visual function in humans. On the one hand, monkeys show considerable return of both elementary and complex visual function, although they typically need intensive and systematic training to overcome the deficit. On the other hand, these experiments show that total and irreversible loss of a particular visual ability is only to be expected if more than one structure of the neural network subserving this ability is injured (for a review, see for example, Frommer, 1978; Rothi & Horner, 1983; Stein, 1994). For example, Mohler and Wurtz (1977) have demonstrated that monkeys no longer recover from blindness after striate cortex injury when their ipsilateral colliculus superior is also destroyed. Similarly, patients with injury to the striate cortex and to the posterior thalamus may show a poorer treatment outcome concerning the compensation of their visual field defect than do patients with injury to the striate cortex only (Zihl, 1995a,b; see p. 59 for further discussion). Thus, the accurate control of the size of the lesion is a crucial issue in studying recovery of vision after brain injury.

The first and foremost question in rehabilitation after brain injury is whether there is any potential at all for recovery. If a particular visual function depends entirely on one single cortical structure, and if this structure is completely and irreversibly injured, then recovery of the affected visual function cannot be expected. Unfortunately, the definition of reversibility and irreversibility of brain injury is still an open issue, despite enormous improvements in brain imaging techniques. In cases of spontaneous recovery it is, of course, reasonable to assume that brain injury merely had reversible consequences (see Bosley et al., 1987). But does the opposite also always hold true, namely that the brain structure in question has really undergone irreversible injury when no spontaneous recovery occurs? A further similarly difficult, but important, question concerns the cortical representation of visual functions. "Functional specialisation" does not imply strict localisation of function. If it did, then injury to a particular cortical area would destroy the function in question completely and irreversibly.

However, the situation is yet more complicated, as the two following case studies will demonstrate.

LM had lost most of her capacity to see motion following bilateral posterior brain injury due to sinus venous thrombosis (Zihl, von Cramon, & Mai, 1983; Zihl, von Cramon, Mai, & Schmid, 1991). She reported, however, to somehow "see" objects in motion, provided that (1) only one stimulus was moving; (2) the speed of the moving stimulus did not exceed 6deg/sec; and (3) objects were moving either horizontally or vertically. This "residual" perception of movement could either constitute incomplete injury to V5 (the "motion" area) or could be accounted for by other visual areas. The measurement of brain activity during the processing of moving visual stimuli in LM showed no evidence of activation of V5 in either hemisphere. Somewhat surprisingly, activation was observed in another visual area (V3) and in the superior parietal cortex (Brodmann's area 7). Both areas, however, are not known to be "functionally specialised" to process visual motion signals and are not activated in normal subjects in the same experimental conditions, but are the likely candidates for the patient's residual movement vision (Shipp et al., 1994). Thus, movement vision is possible without V5, although under extremely restricted conditions. This "residual" movement capacity did not improve over the years and could not be used by LM to substitute the role of her lesioned V5 which would have reduced her severe daily visual handicaps. Nevertheless LM has learned over the years to cope quite successfully with her severe visual disorder. She is able to manage by herself shopping, using public transportation means, keeping her flat and participating in social events as for example birthday parties. Her coping strategies are, however, mainly based on avoiding seeing objects or people in motion.

DF, a patient reported by Milner et al. (1991), suffered a severe visual deficit of form recognition following bilateral posterior brain injury due to asphyxia while taking a shower as a result of a faulty gas water heater. She had great difficulties in discriminating, for example, simple shapes and line orientations. Despite poor performance in these tasks, the patient had little difficulty in everyday visually guided activities such as opening doors, shaking hands, eating meals, reaching out accurately for and grasping objects differing in form, size, and orientation. The authors hypothesised that the preserved visuomotor ability may depend on routes still functioning from the occipital lobe, where the analysis of visual forms is performed, to neural mechanisms in the parietal lobe that control visually guided movements of the hand and fingers. Explicit visual form perception and recognition is therefore not a crucial prerequisite for an appropriate visual guidance for moving hand and fingers. In contrast to LM, who did not benefit from her residual visual motion perception, DF certainly could make use of her "residual" visual form-processing capacity regarding daily life activities.

Certainly, nobody would interpret the use of spared or substituted visual functions in these two cases as recovery, but these and similar observations underline the need for an accurate and detailed analysis of lost, impaired, spared, and substituted visual functions. Otherwise sparing or substitution of function could easily be confounded with recovery of function, especially if practice is required to reveal a spared or substituted visual capacity. Practice might be especially important in cases with denial of preserved vision (so-called negative Anton syndrome), and in cases with a reduction of initiative and self-generated activities due to concomitant depression or reduced motivation (e.g. Feibel & Springer, 1982; Richards & Ruff, 1989). The site and extent of a brain lesion differ, of course, among patients, but this may not be reflected by the (initial) severity of a single visual deficit or pattern of deficits. Recovery of visual function as well as functional improvement through compensation may, however, depend on the integrity of brain structures beyond the visual cortex and on fibre pathways interconnecting the various visual structures. Another difficulty arises because patients cannot (and must not) be kept in a "controlled" constant environment as animals can. Consequently, any kind of improvement of function can also be attributed to confounding "environmental" variables. Finally, how much time should a brain function be given to recover "spontaneously", and how long should treatment be continued before one can reliably state that no (further) improvement can be expected? If systematic intervention is started at an early point in time and the function in question returns, partially or completely, a legitimate explanation would be that the improvement might just as well have taken place without systematic intervention. This is a serious argument, but not easy to dismiss—even if treatment is started several weeks or even months after the onset of a functional deficit and the deficit could therefore be assumed to be stable. One possibility of avoiding this problem is to use a control group to monitor the effect in the experimental group. This seems to be an ideal methodological approach, but again one is forced to deal with the problem of homogeneity of brain injury and the control of environmental influences. Of course, for the patient it is irrelevant why improvement has taken place as long as the outcome is beneficial; for the researcher it is not. There is agreement that the adoption of a method of treatment should be based on an underlying theoretical rationale and on the control for non-specific factors (e.g. motivation, emotional state, social support; Robertson, 1994). These factors may affect or enhance the improvement, although they have little or nothing to do with specific treatment procedures. It seems, therefore, that rehabilitation research in neuropsychology is not only a very laborious and difficult task, for which no really satisfactory methodology exists. At the same time it is also extremely risky because success cannot be guaranteed, even after a high expenditure of time, resources, and energy. However, reports on negative findings are just as important as reports on positive outcomes (Barlow & Hersen, 1985), not only on methodological grounds, but also for extracting criteria on which to base a valid decision about the efficacy of a particular treatment procedure. Of course, when developing and proving new methods of practice, one cannot always predict the potential significance to rehabilitation. What is possible, however, is to design a priori the development and evaluation of treatment methods, to decide on patient eligibility criteria, and to select measures of outcome in the context of behavioural benefit (Baddeley, Meade, & Newcombe, 1980). This is not only important from the viewpoint of rehabilitation, which implies functional improvements for the sake of more independence and higher quality of life, but also for the motivation of patients. The earlier the patient is aware of an improvement in everyday life activities, the higher will be their motivation to co-operate and the earlier the patient will become an expert for the specific individual difficulties, and how to cope with new, unknown and unfamiliar conditions.

Although the number of publications on neuropsychological rehabilitation is increasing and a special journal has been founded for this discipline in 1991 (*Neuropsychological Rehabilitation*), this field still has not been the focus of neuroscientific research. This is a pity because the study of the recovery of brain function and of mechanisms of substitution and compensation is not only of importance for neuropsychological rehabilitation, but also can contribute substantially to the understanding of the functional organisation and reorganisation of the brain and of brain plasticity. The better we understand the relationships between brain and behaviour, especially in "pathological" conditions, the more success we shall have in the development of rehabilitation methods, and the more the patient will benefit. Concerning visual deficits following brain injury, there is meanwhile agreement that rehabilitation is important because vision probably represents the most important sensory system in humans and is required for the guidance of many motor activities. Thus the understanding and accurate identification of visual deficits and the implementation of specific treatment strategies is important to maximise functional independence of patients (Anderson & Rizzo, 1995; Raymond, Bennett, Malia, & Bewick, 1996).

This book deals with the rehabilitation of visual deficits after acquired brain injury. In the following chapters the main cerebral visual disorders will be described, observations of spontaneous recoveries reported, and methods of treatment outlined. To facilitate understanding, each section will begin with a brief description of the particular visual deficit(s) or disorder(s), and consequences for the patient in terms of disability and handicap. Observations of spontaneous recoveries and the rationale and outcome of studies on the effect of treatment will follow. Many observations stem from investigations of the author; some of them have been published, others have not. For some fields of treatment, results of larger groups of patients were available; for others, observations of single cases are presented. Some of the studies, for example on visual field disorders, were systematically prepared and the methodology applied fulfils, at least in part, the criteria required for such studies. Where a sufficiently large number of patients was available, a within-subject repeated-measures design was used, which permits the direct comparison of pre- and post-treatment performance in a given test for each patient. This design is easier to carry out in the context of rehabilitation research than randomised groups studies, and in addition it is similarly effective in demonstrating treatment effects, as shown for example in visual neglect rehabilitation (cf. Antonucci et al., 1995; Pizzamiglio et al., 1993). In other cases, e.g. dyschromatopsia, Balint's syndrome, and visual agnosia, methods of treatment had to be developed *ad hoc* because patients with a disorder sought remediation in order to regain a "critical minimum" of autonomy in their everyday lives, but no proven method of treatment was available. However, even in these cases precautions were taken to differentiate between spontaneous recovery, the effect of treatment, and other, unspecific factors that might also contribute to the observed improvement. In this respect, some of the treatment approaches reported are provisional, and have the character of pilot studies. There is no doubt a great need for developing appropriate and methodologically sound assessment and treatment methods, but hopefully the observations reported here will have some heuristic value for improving and developing such methods and will thus stimulate further research on this issue. It should be mentioned here that the recording of eye movements was a very useful tool to assess a patient's adaptation and compensation behaviour in scanning and searching tasks as well as in reading. In addition, it allowed the precise measurement of saccadic localisation performance and fixation accuracy. Furthermore, the analysis of eye movements before and after practice enabled us to measure and understand the adaptive processes underlying the observed improvements. Eye movements can therefore be used to objectively assess practice effects. Interestingly enough, patients were highly interested to know about their eye movements during reading and scanning, and were then quite surprised to learn how laborious and time-consuming their eye movement guidance was. The demonstration of the eye movement recordings allowed us to better explain to the patient not only her or his very individual disorder, but also why treatment is needed and how practice will be constructed. This information may well have supported patients' insight into their visual deficits and may also have increased the motivation for the treatment required. It was a great concern and at the same time a challenge for us to make every patient an expert of her or his visual difficulties and problems.

A special section is devoted to patients suffering from central scotoma. Although this visual field disorder is a rare condition, these patients typically show a combination of severe visual deficits and therefore need special rehabilitation measures.

CHAPTER TWO

Visual field disorders

FORMS AND FREQUENCY OF OCCURRENCE

Visual field disorders can result from injury to the visual pathway anywhere between the retina and the striate cortex. The site of decussation of the retinogeniculate fibres, the optic chiasm, is used as an anatomical landmark to differentiate between the prechiasmatic or peripheral and the postchiasmatic (retrochiasmatic) or central visual pathway. While unilateral injury to the pre-chiasmatic pathway affects the ipsilesional field only, postchiasmatic injury causes visual deficits in both monocular hemifields contralateral to the site of injury. The resulting field disorders are therefore referred to as "homonymous" (for reviews, see Harrington, 1976; Miller, 1982; Walsh & Hoyt, 1969). Visual field disorders can be measured quantitatively by perimetric techniques (see, e.g. Aulhorn & Harms, 1972; Ellenberger, 1974; Harrington, 1976). In clinical routine perimetry, a light target of a given size and luminance is slowly moved from the periphery towards the centre of the perimetric sphere. The subject's task is to detect the target and to indicate its appearance by pressing a buzzer-key, while he or she is steadily fixating a small red dot in the centre of the perimeter. The extent of the visual field is defined by those positions where the target is detected by the subject. Detailed perimetric testing also comprises the mapping of the field for colour and form targets, thus allowing a qualitative and quantitative characterisation of vision in every portion of the visual field.

Homonymous field disorders are usually classified according to (1) the quality of the deficit; (2) the portion of the field affected; and (3) the quantitative extent of the deficit. Concerning the quality of the disorder, vision can either be completely lost in the affected field region (anopia), or one or more but not all visual functions can be affected. For example, light vision may be preserved but depressed, while colour and form vision are lost (so-called cerebral amblyopia),

11

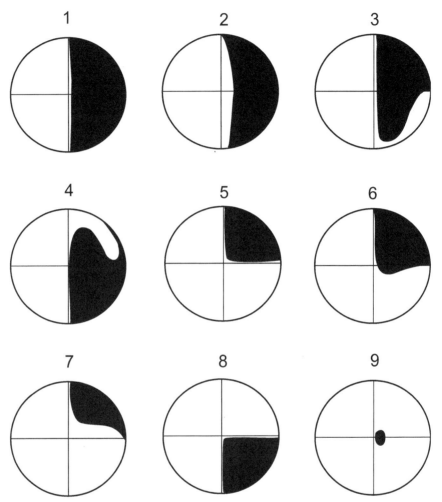

FIG. 2.1   Examples of unilateral homonymous field loss (affected binocular regions in black). 1, 2: hemianopia with foveal (1.5°) or macular (6°) sparing; 3, 4: hemianopia with sparing of the temporal crescent ("half moon") in the lower or upper hemifield; 5, 6, 7: upper quadranopia with varying degrees of sparing; 8: lower quadranopia; 9: paracentral scotoma.

or colour vision can be lost while other visual functions are preserved (achromatopsia). Figures 2.1–2.3 show the most frequent forms of homonymous visual field disorders after uni- and bilateral brain injury. The most common type is hemianopia (loss of vision in one hemifield), followed by quadranopia (loss of vision in one quadrant), and paracentral scotoma (island of blindness in the parafoveal field region). Homonymous amblyopia typically affects one hemifield (hemiamblyopia), while selective loss of colour vision can be found in the hemifield (hemiachromatopsia) as well as in the upper quadrant.

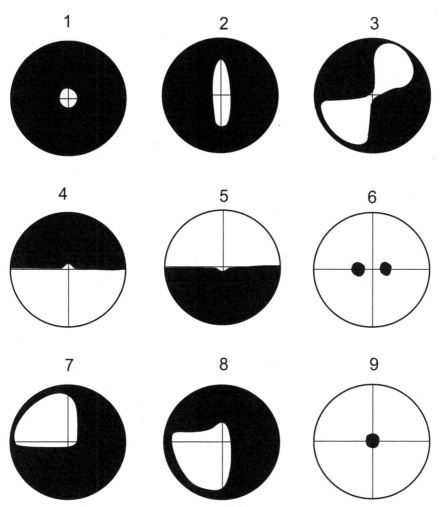

FIG. 2.2 Examples of bilateral homonymous field loss (affected binocular regions in black). 1: bilateral hemianopia ("tunnel vision"); 2: bilateral hemianopia with sparing along the upper and lower vertical axes; 3: bilateral crossed quadranopia; 4, 5: bilateral upper (superior) and lower (inferior) hemianopia; 6: bilateral paracentral scotomata; 7, 8: loss of three quadrants; 9: central scotoma.

Table 2.1 summarises the most common forms of homonymous visual field disorders, their frequency of occurrence, and the underlying aetiology. Unilateral homonymous visual field disorders are much more frequent (about 90%) than bilateral homonymous field disorders. Concerning aetiology, stroke represents the most common type (about 60%) of brain injury (see also Trobe, Lorber, & Schlezinger, 1973; Zihl, 1989). Visual field sparing, on the one hand, refers to

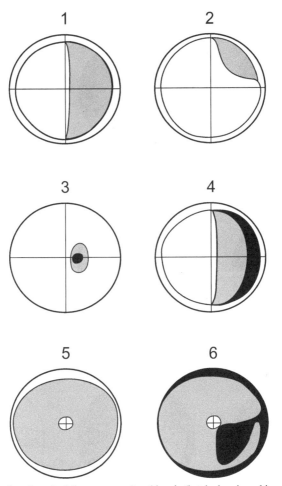

FIG. 2.3 Examples of cerebral (homonymous) amblyopia (hatched regions; binocular testing conditions). 1: hemiamblyopia; 2: incomplete upper amblyopia; 3: amblyopic region around a paracentral scotoma; 4: hemiamblyopia with loss of temporal crescent; 5: bilateral hemiamblyopia with central sparing; 6: bilateral amblyopia with incomplete lower quadranopia and partial sparing of the temporal crescent. Black areas indicate total loss of vision.

the portion of the visual field where vision is preserved, i.e. a hemifield, a quadrant, etc., and on the other hand, it also refers to the extent of sparing in the affected hemifield, expressed in degrees of visual angle (°) measured from the fovea. As Table 2.2 shows, in the majority of patients field sparing varies between 0.5° and 5°. As a rule, patients with small visual field sparing are more disabled, especially with regard to visual abilities that crucially depend on the parafoveal region, such as reading (see p. 72).

TABLE 2.1

Homonymous visual field disorders in
714 patients with postchiasmatic
brain injury: Types and aetiology

Type and aetiology	n	%
(A) Type of field defect		
Unilateral (n = 634; 88.8%)		
Hemianopia	413	65.2
Upper quadranopia	54	8.5
Lower quadranopia	48	7.6
Paracentral scotoma	49	7.7
Hemiamblyopia	70	11.0
Bilateral (n = 80; 11.2%)		
Hemianopia	43	53.8
Quadranopia (upper and lower)	8	10.0
Paracentral scotoma	11	13.7
Central scotoma	10	12.5
Amblyopia	8	10.0
(B) Aetiology		
Occipital stroke	439	61.5
Occipital haemorrhage	104	14.6
Closed head trauma	81	11.3
Tumour (operated)	39	5.5
Hypoxia	28	3.9
Others	23	3.2

TABLE 2.2

Visual field sparing in patients with unilateral field disorders
(n = 634; numbers refer to percentages)

Type of defect	< 2°	2–4°	5–10°	> 10°
Hemianopia (n = 413)	34.1	40.3	18.0	7.6
Upper quadranopia (n = 54)	18.2	40.2	28.4	13.2
Lower quadranopia (n = 48)	16.7	37.5	29.2	16.6
Paracentral scotoma (n = 49)	34.7	38.8	22.5	4.0
Hemiamblyopia (n = 70)	31.5	34.3	23.9	10.2

SPONTANEOUS RECOVERY

It has been known for a long time that vision can return in patients with uni- and
bilateral postchiasmatic injury, but only few systematic studies on a larger group
of cases exist. Hier, Mondlock, and Caplan (1983b) found recovery in about
30% of 41 patients with unilateral homonymous field loss within up to about 8

months. These authors used confrontation testing instead of quantitative perimetry and coded recovery in terms of presence or absence of hemianopia. In a group of 111 patients with unilateral field loss, we (Zihl & von Cramon, 1986a) observed spontaneous recovery in 12% of the patients. A similar percentage (16%) was found within the first 3 months in a group of 225 patients with unilateral visual field loss (Zihl, 1994). Interestingly, recovery was smaller (mean = 3°; range = 1–6°) in patients with visual field sparing of less than 5°, as compared to patients with at least 10° of sparing (mean = 7°; range = 3–24°). Complete spontaneous recovery from hemianopia was observed in only four cases (1.8%), all of which had suffered from occipital haemorrhage. Figure 2.4 shows examples of spontaneous visual field recovery. Concerning the quality of vision in field regions that recovered from blindness, light vision typically is followed by colour and form vision. In some cases the recovered field region may remain amblyopic, i.e. only light vision returns, and even this visual function may remain depressed. It should be added here that spontaneous recovery from homonymous hemianopia has also been observed in patients suffering from multiple sclerosis (for a review, see McDonald & Barnes, 1992). Plant et al. (1992) found complete recovery in 14 out of 18 patients within 4 weeks to 12 months. However, hemianopia may also persist as a chronic deficit in multiple sclerosis.

Spontaneous recovery of vision has also been reported in patients suffering from complete cerebral blindness. Summarising the observations reported by various authors (Bergmann, 1957; Gloning, Gloning, & Tschabitscher, 1962; Symonds & Mackenzie, 1957) on a total of 111 patients, 81 patients (73%) showed recovery of vision, with the time course and the extent of recovery varying considerably. Complete recovery was found in only 6% of cases; the rest showed partial recovery of vision. Recovery of vision normally occurred within 8 to 12 weeks; however, in some patients recovery has been observed up to 2 years after brain injury. The pattern of return of vision was found to follow more or less definite stages (Gloning et al., 1962; Poppelreuter, 1917/1990; Teuber et al., 1960). Light perception recovers first, often as an undifferentiated sensation which can be elicited much more easily when flickering or moving stimuli are used. The patients are usually unable to indicate the direction or speed of movement, but can often report the location of the stimulus. At the next stage, patients may report "vague" impressions of contours; vision is typically "foggy", and visual acuity may be reduced to finger counting. Colours may appear pale or at least less saturated than previously. Vision may further improve to a degree that the patient can visually recognise objects, faces, and surroundings. As a rule, vision returns in the central field regions; there are, however, also cases with recovery of vision in the peripheral visual field only (Symonds & Mackenzie, 1957). The extent of recovery of vision in patients with complete cerebral blindness in the acute stage was found to be negatively correlated with aetiology (spontaneous stroke), time elapsed since brain injury, and a history of diabetes or hypertension (Aldrich, Alessi, Beck, & Gilman, 1987).

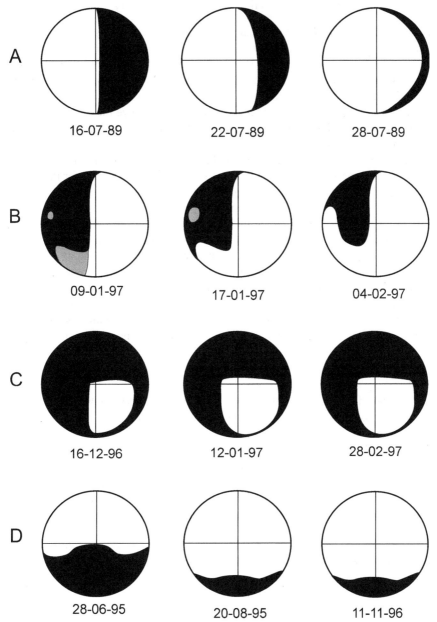

FIG. 2.4 Spontaneous return of visual field (binocular field plots) in four patients with either uni- (A, B) or bilateral (C, D) homonymous field loss (60° plots) after occipital stroke. Black areas: regions of lost vision; grey areas: amblyopic regions. Dates below field plots indicate times of perimetric testing.

SPONTANEOUS ADAPTATION

Since sufficient spontaneous visual field recovery can be expected only in a small group of patients, the question arises as to which means are available to all other patients to overcome their visual impairment. The most obvious solution is to substitute the lost field region by gaze shifts. Head movements are usually guided by the size and temporal course of saccadic eye movements (Uemura, Arai, & Shimazaki, 1980); thus the "natural" sequence is that eye movements precede head movements. Reversing this order affects the eye–head co-ordination in hemianopia patients (Zangemeister, Meienberg, Stark, & Hoyt, 1982) and impairs visual exploration (Kerkhoff et al., 1992b). Consequently, the use of eye movements appears to be the appropriate means of compensating for the visual field loss. Since eye movements represent a patient's own means of substituting the lost field region, one could assume that patients spontaneously make use of this means. This form of adaptation can be expected all the more because the visual field defect restricts a patient's overview and impairs simultaneous perception and spatial orientation. As a result, comprehending a scene or a word as a whole, detecting obstacles on the affected side and avoiding people approaching from that side and finding one's way may become difficult. Such experiences should make the patient aware of the visual field loss and may "force" the more frequent use of gaze shifts to overcome the various handicaps. Although this argumentation appears sensible and is, for example, supported by the observations reported by Gassel and Williams (1963a,b), patients are not always aware of their visual defect and do not use eye shifts to compensate effectively for their field loss.

Critchley (1949) identified various degrees of awareness and unawareness, respectively, of patients with visual field defects:

(1) Total lack of awareness of the defect.
(2) Unawareness of the defect itself, but a recognition of the consequences of the defect (e.g. frequent bumping into persons or objects on one side without knowing why).
(3) "Projection" of the defect, i.e. rationalising it as being due to, e.g. imperfect illumination.
(4) Realisation that there is "something wrong" with vision, although the nature of the defect is not understood, nor can it be described.
(5) Awareness of a visual defect to one side, misinterpreted as a defect of vision in one eye.
(6) Full awareness of the hemianopia defect.

As Critchley further pointed out, posterior lesions in the visual system are more often associated with an impaired awareness than more anteriorly located lesions, an observation that has been supported by Koehler, Endtz, Te Velde, and Hekster

(1986). However, "awareness" of a deficit is not simply a question of insight into the deficit in the sense of cognitive elaboration. Although many patients show mental confusion in the acute stage of brain injury, and the absence of awareness with respect to the field defect may be explained by this, lack of awareness may still persist after mental confusion has disappeared. In search for an explanation, Levine (1990) suggested that injury to the visual pathway (as well as to other sensory pathways) at any level is not necessarily associated with any immediate sensory experience that uniquely specifies the defect. Thus, a field defect is not automatically accompanied by specific information about and hence direct experience of the absence of vision in that particular field region. Instead, the visual loss must be discovered by the subject through a process of self-observation and inference. Therefore it is not surprising that unawareness of the field defect is a common phenomenon even in patients with normal intellectual functions. Due to the absence of an immediate sensation, a hemianopic patient has to infer the visual deficit from failures resulting from it, i.e. from visual experience. Since detection and awareness of visual loss require curiosity, self-observation, inference, and memory, a variety of neuropsychological deficits may interfere with and thereby impair the acquisition of knowledge about failures resulting from visual loss. In addition to cognitive abilities and motivation, personality may also play a role. As Levine (1990) mentioned, discovery of visual loss requires the "ability to change the mental set or outlook based on evidence from the external world". Awareness of visual loss may thus also depend on cognitive flexibility. Individuals with a rather rigid personality are therefore more likely to trust their own explanation(s) of their visual loss than relate their failures to their visual defect, and may not use their experiences to discover the real cause of their everyday difficulties. However, the presence of awareness does not necessarily imply that the patient effectively compensates for the visual field loss. Effective compensation undoubtedly implies knowledge of how to compensate. However, as will be discussed later (p. 59), (spontaneous) compensation also depends on the preservation of subcortical and cortical fibre connections (Zihl, 1995a,b).

It was Poppelreuter (1917/1990) who first reported cases with remarkable oculomotor compensation of field loss; 7 out of 28 (25%) of his patients successfully substituted their lost visual field by appropriate eye movement strategies. Gassel and Williams (1963a,b) also found an "extraordinary ability" to compensate for hemianopia in the majority of their 35 patients, and attributed the adjustment to the field defect to a shift in the "straight ahead" and thus of attention to the hemianopic side, as well as to the use of occasional "abrupt" saccadic gaze shifts towards that side. Interestingly, the spontaneous use of compensatory strategies did not depend on whether a patient had full insight into his field defect or not. Gassel and Williams (1963b) have hypothesised that patients do not realise the presence of their field loss, because the eye movements and changes in attention towards the affected side "are made so rapidly".

Possibly their well-timed gaze shifts re-established the (temporal and spatial) coherence of successive visual impressions, which in turn let the patient experience "seeing" the visual surroundings at "one glance". In contrast to these positive observations, Poppelreuter (1917/1990) noted that the majority of his patients used a less efficient oculomotor compensation strategy. For the assessment of visual scanning impairments, he developed (p. 105; Fig. 2.5) "an exact method, including the measurement of time, standardised for all patients" to map the field of search. Numbers, letters, and figures (rectangles, circles, semicircles, crosses, and triangles) in the colours red, green, blue, yellow, and black were presented on a white board, 1m^2 in size, fitted into a black wooden frame behind a glass plate. In total, 57 items were distributed in an irregular but evenly spaced array over the board; 30 items were selected for the visual search test. The patient sat in a chair at a distance of 0.5m in front of the board. After the name of an item was called out the patient had to open his eyes, search for the object, and touch it immediately with a stick (an old-fashioned but effective version of a touch screen). Poppelreuter measured the time a patient required to search for the target, and also assessed the quality of the search strategy, i.e. whether the patient searched for the target in a systematic or an irregular way. Apart from cases with occipital injuries, Poppelreuter also tested a group of normal subjects ($n = 20$) and a group of soldiers with cranial gunshots ($n = 22$) sparing posterior brain structures. Searching times for these two groups were less than 9.8sec; Poppelreuter therefore classified patients with search times of 10sec or longer as impaired in visual search. In the group of patients with homonymous hemianopia ($n = 14$) eight subjects performed normally; mean search time of the cases with impaired visual search was 17.1sec (range = 10.5–24.3sec). In the group with bilateral field defects ($n = 12$), five patients performed within the range of control subjects; the mean search time of the impaired group was 23.5sec (range = 11.9–55.1sec). In addition to increased search times, Poppelreuter observed that patients showed a "characteristic clumsiness": They "allowed their gaze to wander unsystematically" through the stimulus array. Furthermore, saccadic eye movements were "fragmented", i.e. hypometric, and patients used a high number of fixations, resulting in a highly time-consuming and "very laborious" visual search process. The impairment in visual search, however, could not entirely be explained by the visual field defect, because no systematic relationship was found between the severity of the field defect and visual scanning and visual search performance.

Saccadic hypometria was also reported by other authors using electrooculography for the recording of eye movements (Chedru, Leblanc, & Lhermitte, 1973; Meienberg et al., 1981; Williams & Gassel, 1962). Patients with saccadic hypometria have to make several saccades to shift their gaze towards a target and to get a complete view over the hemispace corresponding to the side of visual field loss. As a consequence, patients may omit objects or parts of the visual surroundings located on the affected side, or at least require more time for

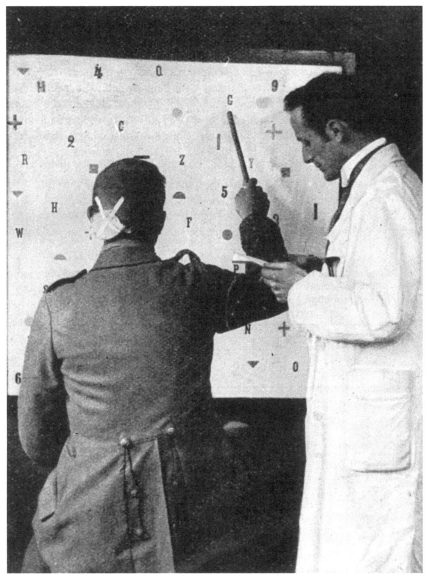

FIG. 2.5 Poppelreuter (right) testing a patient with field loss for his visual searching ability (from W. Poppelreuter, *Disturbances of lower and higher visual capacities caused by occipital damage*, 1917/1990, p. 106. With permission of Oxford University Press).

its exploration (Ishiai, Furkawa, & Tsukagoshi, 1987). In a typical everyday situation, for example in a supermarket or a crowded place, the slowness of visual exploration and the impaired simultaneous overview may represent a serious impairment. Patients may bump into objects on one side and may even neglect people or obstacles on their "good" side when shifting their gaze totally to the affected side (Gassel & Williams, 1963b).

To further elucidate spontaneous oculomotor compensation we analysed the eye movements in a total of 166 patients with homonymous uni- and bilateral visual field loss due to occipital lobe injury (for clinical details, see Tables 2.3A, B, & C). Patients did not show additional disturbances in the anterior visual pathways or of the oculomotor system, as detailed ophthalmologic examination revealed. (Corrected) monocular visual acuity (Snellen fraction) was at least 0.90 for near and far vision. According to the criteria proposed by Halligan, Cockburn, and Wilson (1991), patients did not exhibit symptoms of visual neglect, when tested on visual search, letter cancellation, figure and shape copying, line (length 30cm) bisection, "representational drawing" (drawing from memory), text reading, and reading of numbers (2–6 characters). Eye movements

TABLE 2.3A

Clinical details of a group of 166 patients (104 males, 62 females) with uni- or bilateral homonymous field disorders who were examined for oculomotor compensation (mean time since brain injury was 9 weeks, range = 4–28 weeks). Aetiology and age

	CV	TBI	Tumour (operated)
Cases	104 (62.7%)	52 (31.3%)	10 (6.0%)
Age (median and range)	57 (23–85)	27 (16–42)	35 (24–43)

CV: cerebrovascular disease; TBI: traumatic brain injury.

TABLE 2.3B

Type of field deficit (patients as in Table 2.3A)

Defect	Left-sided	Right-sided
Unilateral (n = 130)		
Hemianopia	52	38
Upper quadranopia	7	7
Lower quadranopia	2	5
Paracentral scotoma	3	2
Hemiamblyopia	7	7
Bilateral (n = 36)		
Hemianopia	10	
Quadranopia	2	
Paracentral scotoma	5	
Hemiamblyopia	13	
Central scotoma	6	

TABLE 2.3C
Visual field sparing (percentages in brackets. Patients as in Table 2.3A)

Defect	1–2°	< = 3°	3–5°	4–5°	> 5°	6–10°	> 10°
Unilateral							
Hemianopia	50 (55.6)	–	26 (28.8)	–	–	7 (7.8)	7 (7.8)
Quadranopia	4 (19.0)	–	12 (63.2)	–	–	4 (19.0)	1 (1.2)
Paracentral scotoma	5	–	–	–	–	–	–
Hemiamblyopia*	7	–	5	–	–	2	–
Bilateral**							
Hemianopia	–	1	–	4	5	–	–
Paracentral scotoma	–	3	–	2	–	–	–
Hemiamblyopia	–	6	–	4	3	–	–
Central scotoma***	–	–	–	4	2	–	–

*sparing of form field; **mean diameter of spared central field; ***mean diameter of scotoma.

were recorded using the pupil-corneal-reflection method (Young & Sheena, 1975). The eye movement recording system consisted of a microprocessor system (Debic 84, Demel, Haan, Germany) connected to a video system. The dominant eye was illuminated by infrared light, and the reflections were recorded and used to calculate the fixation positions every 20msec in terms of x- and y-positions. Two stimulus conditions (see Fig. 2.6) were used to assess visually guided oculomotor scanning behaviour: saccadic accuracy and oculomotor scanning. In the first testing condition we asked patients to alternately shift their fixation with one sweep between two small light spots in the horizontal plane (horizontal saccade condition). The distance between the two stimuli was 20°, their diameter was 0.9°. In the second testing condition (oculomotor scanning condition), an irregular pattern of 20 dots (diameter: 0.9°) was used. Display size was 40° horizontally, and 32° vertically. Dot luminance was 27cd/m^2; background luminance was 0.2cd/m^2. The minimal spatial separation of the dots in the scanning condition was 7° (range = 4.3–10.5°). To avoid cues from the surroundings, room illumination was kept very low (1 lux). Subjects were asked to count the dots presented on a screen, but no instruction was given on the number of dots or how to proceed with counting or searching. This test is similar to the dot cancellation test (Lezak, 1995) but did not include feedback on which dots have already been processed. Eye movement recording in the scanning condition was started with the onset of dot pattern presentation and was ended when the subject indicated to have counted all dots. Eye movements were analysed with respect to hypometria in the horizontal saccade condition and with respect to fixations and saccades in the oculomotor scanning condition. A fixation was defined as eye rest for at least 120msec within a window of 1.5° in diameter, which is well beyond the amplitudes of microsaccades, microdrift, or microtremor (Leigh & Zee, 1991).

A

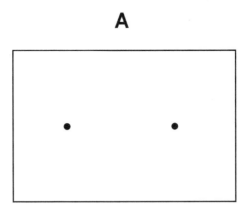

B

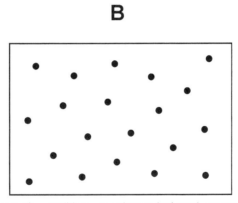

FIG. 2.6 Oculomotor testing conditions. A: voluntary horizontal eye movements (distance between targets: 20°); B: visual scanning (20 dots).

In the horizontal saccade condition, eye movements were recorded in 145 patients. The majority of patients ($n = 125$) suffered from unilateral field disorders, 20 patients showed bilateral field disorders. Mean field sparing was 2.2° (SD = 0.9) in the group with left-sided hemianopia ($n = 52$), and 2.4° (SD = 1.1) in the group with right-sided hemianopia ($n = 38$). Mean diameter of preserved visual field in the group with bilateral field disorders ($n = 20$) was 14.6° (range = 8–19°). Time since lesion was on average 18.4 weeks (range = 5–27). Figure 2.7 shows examples of voluntary horizontal eye movements in normal subjects and in patients with uni- and bilateral homonymous field defects. Saccadic gain was used to characterise saccadic accuracy and was calculated as the quotient of

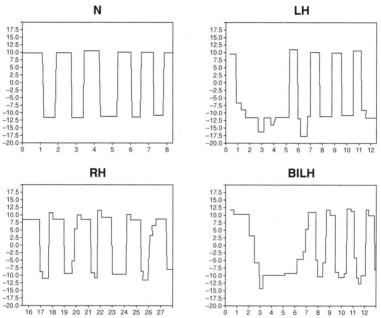

FIG. 2.7 Voluntary horizontal eye movements in a normal subject (N), a patient with left-sided hemianopia (LH; sparing = 2°), a patient with a right-sided hemianopia (RH; field sparing = 3°), and a patient with bilateral hemianopia (BILH; diameter of spared central field = 8°). Bottom: left, top: right. x-axis: time period of recording (in sec); y-axis: horizontal amplitude (in degrees) of saccades (0 = centre). Note hypometria but also hypermetria of saccades especially to the affected side.

initial saccadic amplitude and target distance. A saccadic gain of 1 indicates perfect correspondence between target and eye position. In the group with uni-lateral hemianopia, 64 out of 90 patients (71%) showed dysmetria; bilateral field loss affected saccadic accuracy in all patients (see Table 2.4). The percentage of cases with dysmetric saccades to the affected side was nearly equal in both left- (73%) and right-sided (68%) hemianopic groups; the side of brain injury was therefore not a crucial factor. In addition, saccadic dysmetria was also found for saccades directed to the ipsilateral ("good") hemifield. Saccadic dysmetria became typically apparent in the form of hypometric saccades; only about one quarter (25.6%) of hemianopic patients showed hypermetric saccades to the affected side, i.e. their saccades exceeded the position of the target. Patients with upper or lower quadranopia, or with hemiamblyopia, also showed hypometric saccades towards the contralateral (i.e. defective) side and hypermetric saccades towards the ipsilateral side. Patients with bilateral field disorders mainly showed hypometric saccades to both sides. To sum up, the majority of patients with uni- and bilateral field loss use eye movements which are too small to compensate effectively for the field loss. As a consequence, these patients may require a

TABLE 2.4

Accuracy of saccades to the left and to the right ($n = 10$ each; amplitudes, in degrees, and gain) in patients with uni- and bilateral field disorders. Visual field sparing did not exceed 10°

	Direction	Normal	Hypometric	Hypermetric
LH ($n = 52$)	←	14	26	12
	→	24	16	12
RH ($n = 38$)	←	20	8	10
	→	12	15	11
LQ ($n = 9$)	←	4	3	2
	→	5	3	1
RQ ($n = 12$)	←	8	1	3
	→	7	2	3
LHA ($n = 7$)	←	4	2	1
	→	5	0	2
RHA ($n = 7$)	←	6	0	1
	→	5	2	0
BILH ($n = 7$)	←	0	5	2
	→	0	4	3
BILHA ($n = 13$)	←	3	5	5
	→	4	6	3

LH: patients with left-sided hemianopia; RH: patients with right-sided hemianopia; LQ, RQ: patients with left- and right-sided upper or lower quadranopia; LHA, RHA patients with left- and right-sided hemiamblyopia; BILH: patients with bilateral hemianopia; BILHA: patients with bilateral amblyopia. Patients were classified as "normal" when their gain was in the range of 25 normal subjects (i.e. between 0.95 and 1.05), as "hypometric" when the gain was < 0.95, and as "hypermetric" when the gain was > 1.05). ←, →: saccades to the left and to the right, respectively. Numbers refer to number of patients.

FIG. 2.8 (opposite) Oculomotor scanning patterns during the scanning of a dot pattern (see Fig. 2.6B) in normal subjects (N1, N2) and in patients with unilateral homonymous field disorders with (+) and without (−) effective spontaneous oculomotor compensation at time of first testing. Abbreviations: LH, RH: left- and right-sided hemianopia; LUQ: left upper quadranopia; LHA: left-sided hemiamblyopia; LPCS: left-sided paracentral scotoma. Scanning times (in sec): N1: 7.4, N2: 11.9; LH+ (3° sparing; 6 weeks post-injury): 10.1; LH- (2°; 8 weeks): 20.1; RH+ (1°; 7 weeks): 11.2; RH- (1°; 7 weeks): 17.9; LUQ+ (3°; 6 weeks): 11.8; LUQ- (5°; 9 weeks): 15.9; LHA+ (3°; 6 weeks): 11.3; LHA- (2°; 7 weeks): 15.3; LPCS+ (1°; 8 weeks): 8.8; LPCS- (2°; 9 weeks): 18.1. Mean scanning time in a group of 30 age-matched normal control subjects was 9.3sec (range = 6.2– 12.8). x-axis: horizontal extension of stimulus array (in degrees; 0 = centre, negative values left, positive values right), y-axis: vertical extension (0 = centre, negative values down, positive values up). Dots indicate fixation locations. All subjects reported correctly 20 dots. Note the increased number of saccades and fixations in "−" patients as compared to normal subjects and "+" patients.

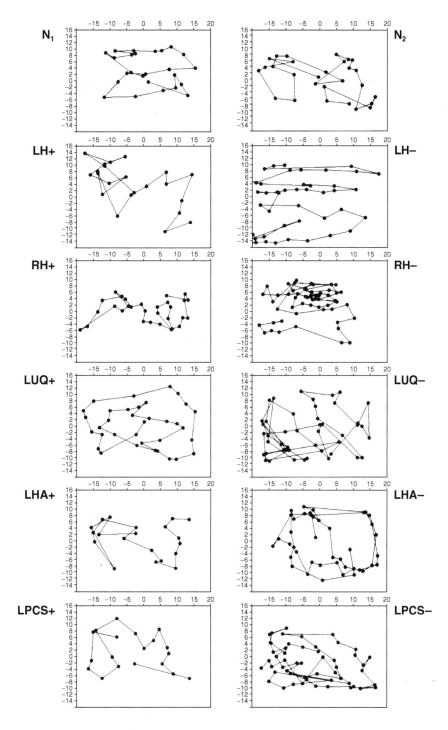

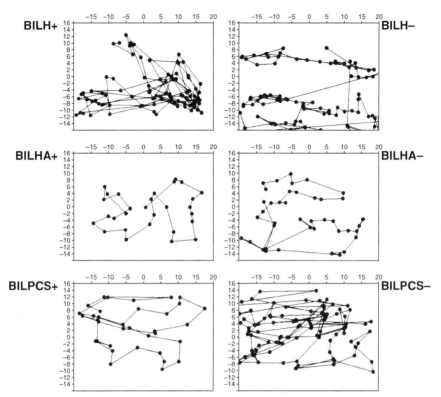

FIG. 2.9   Oculomotor scanning patterns during the scanning of a dot pattern (see Fig. 2.6B) in patients with bilateral homonymous field disorders with (+) and without (−) spontaneous oculomotor compensation at time of first testing. Abbreviations: BILH: bilateral hemianopia; BILHA: bilateral hemiamblyopia; BILPCS: bilateral paracentral scotoma. Scanning times (in sec): BILH+ (8° central field sparing; 11 weeks): 49.1 sec; BILH- (11°; 16 weeks): 98.1; BILHA+ (9°; 8 weeks): 9.1; BILHA- (11°; 11 weeks): 15.8; BILPCS+ (5°; 7 weeks): 13.4; BILPCS- (6°; 8 weeks): 50.7. Both BILHA- patients reported correctly 20 dots; the BILH+ patient reported 16, and the BILH- patient 14 dots. The BILPCS- patients reported 19 and 18 dots, respectively. Further details as in Fig. 2.8.

higher number of saccades to gain a complete view over the visual surroundings, resulting in a considerable increase of scanning time. Under time-restricted viewing conditions there may also be a tendency to neglect part of the surroundings in both the affected and the intact hemifield (see also Gassel & Williams, 1963b). Complaints made by patients about the "slowness" of their vision (cf. Table 2.7 p. 31) may, at least in part, be explained by their hypometric saccades.

The analysis of eye movement patterns during scanning of the dot pattern produced even clearer observations and confirmed, in part, the predictions made on the basis of voluntary horizontal saccades. Figures 2.8 and 2.9 show examples of oculomotor scanning in patients with uni- and bilateral visual field defects. Despite the same side of field loss and the same degree of field sparing, patients differed with respect to their compensatory behaviour, which either was very effective or was characterised by a high number of saccades and fixations. Table 2.5 summarises scanning times in the entire group of patients with uni- and bilateral visual field defects. An upper cut-off scanning time was calculated on the basis of data from 30 age-matched control subjects (mean time = 9.3sec; SD = 0.8; range = 6.4–12.6sec). Patients with a scanning time that was longer than 13sec were classified as "impaired". According to this criterion, all patients with bilateral visual field loss were impaired, 62% of patients with left-sided hemianopia, 60% of patients with right-sided hemianopia, and 48% of patients with quadranopia. Interestingly, patients with left-sided and with right-sided hemianopia showed comparable performance, while patients with lower quadranopia were

TABLE 2.5

Oculomotor scanning times (in seconds) in a dot counting task (Fig. 2.6) in a group of 155 patients with uni- and bilateral visual field defects

	Number of cases	Mean	1SD
LHa	20	9.9	1.3
LHb	32	26.0	6.4
RHa	15	9.6	0.9
RHb	23	24.9	6.5
UQa	9	10.7	1.4
UQb	5	21.1	4.5
LQa	2	9.8	–
LQb	5	25.0	7.3
PSCa	3	9.4	–
PSCb	2	13.2	–
HAa	6	10.6	1.3
HAb	8	15.0	5.1
BILHa	0	–	–
BILHb	7	40.3	9.8
BILPCSa	1	11.4	–
BILPCSb	4	14.9	–
BILHAa	2	11.9	–
BILHAb	11	23.8	7.7
N	30	9.3	0.8

LH: patients with left-sided hemianopia; RH: patients with right-sided hemianopia; UQ: patients with upper quadranopia; LQ: patients with lower quadranopia; PSC: patients with unilateral paracentral scotoma; HA: patients with hemiamblyopia; BILH: patients with bilateral field loss; BILPSC: patients with bilateral paracentral scotoma; BILHA: patients with bilateral amblyopia. a: subgroups with scanning times in the range of normal controls, b: subgroups with elevated scanning times (> 13sec); N: age-matched control subjects for comparison.

more often impaired (5 out of 7) than were patients with upper quadranopia (5 out of 14). Patients with paracentral scotoma also showed elevated scanning times, with bilateral scotoma particularly affecting oculomotor scanning. Hemiamblyopia and bilateral amblyopia also impaired oculomotor scanning, but to a lesser degree than uni- or bilateral hemianopia.

Surprisingly, scanning times of patients with hemi- or quadranopia, and with hemiamblyopia, were not associated with the degree of visual field sparing (cf. Table 2.6) in such a way that the smaller the degree of sparing, the more impaired the oculomotor scanning would be. Visual field sparing *per se* therefore appears not to be a crucial factor for oculomotor scanning performance. This finding is in agreement with Poppelreuter's (1917/1990) observations, and is further supported by the outcome of a recent study (Zihl, 1995b) that showed that complete hemianopia after injury to the optic radiation or to the striate cortex is not necessarily associated with impaired oculomotor scanning. Additional involvement of the posterior thalamus and/or the occipitoparietal cortex, and the reciprocal fibre connections are required for impairment of oculomotor scanning (for further discussion, see p. 59). Thus, the prognosis concerning effective spontaneous adaptation appears worse in patients with additional injury to subcortical and/or occipitoparietal structures (see Dromerick & Reding, 1995, for a different view).

Patients' reports of their visual disability are in close agreement with their oculomotor scanning behaviour, especially in unfamiliar environments. Table 2.7 shows the number of patients with unilateral and bilateral field defects who reported difficulties in everyday life. More than half of the patients (60.8%) with

TABLE 2.6

Oculomotor scanning times (in seconds) in a dot counting task (see Figure 2.6B) and visual field sparing in a group of 111 patients with unilateral homonymous field loss

Sparing		< 2°	3–5°	> 5°
LH (n = 48)	n	25	16	7
	Mean	17.9	15.6	16.5
	1SD	8.8	9.9	6.3
RH (n = 38)	n	22	9	7
	Mean	17.6	17.5	18.1
	1SD	9.0	9.7	8.4
Q (n = 25)	n	8	11	6
	Mean	15.7	19.3	14.7
	1SD	8.7	9.1	3.0
N (n = 30)		9.3 (range = 6.2–12.8)		

LH: patients with left-sided hemianopia; RH: patients with right-sided hemianopia; Q: patients with (upper or lower) quadranopia; N: age-matched normal control subjects.

TABLE 2.7

Report of 145 patients with homonymous visual field loss about difficulties in everyday life in familiar and unfamiliar surroundings, and forms of awareness of field defects

	LH (n = 52) n (%)	RH (n = 38) n (%)	Q (n = 21) n (%)	HA (n = 14) n (%)	BILH (n = 7) n (%)	BILHA (n = 13) n (%)
Vision "too slow"						
Familiar surroundings	6 (11.5)	7 (18.4)	4* (19.1)	2 (14.3)	7 (100)	9 (64.3)
Unfamiliar surroundings	46 (88.5)	31 (81.6)	5* (23.8)	6 (42.9)	7 (100)	13 (100)
Bumping against obstacles						
Familiar surroundings	4 (7.7)	4 (10.5)	2* (9.5)	2 (14.3)	4 (57.1)	4 (30.8)
Unfamiliar surroundings	21 (40.4)	16 (42.1)	5* (23.8)	4 (28.6)	6 (85.7)	6 (46.2)
"Getting lost"						
Familiar surroundings	3 (5.8)	1 (2.6)	1* (4.8)	1 (7.1)	4 (57.1)	3 (23.1)
Unfamiliar surroundings	19 (36.5)	13 (34.2)	2* (9.5)	1 (7.1)	7 (100)	4 (30.8)
Awareness of visual field loss						
Full awareness	10 (19.2)	7 (18.4)	6 (28.6)	8 (57.1)	1 (14.3)	6 (46.2)
"Bad vision"	18 (34.6)	10 (26.3)	9 (42.8)	6 (42.9)	1 (14.3)	7 (53.8)
External factors	7 (13.5)	9 (23.7)	3* (14.3)	0	0	0
No awareness	17 (32.7)	12 (31.6)	3* (14.3)	0	5 (71.4)	0

LH: patients with left-sided hemianopia; RH: patients with right-sided hemianopia; Q: patients with quadranopia; HA: patients with hemiamblyopia; BILH: patients with bilateral hemianopia; BILHA: patients with bilateral amblyopia. *mainly patients with lower quadranopia.

unilateral, and all patients with bilateral visual field disorders reported difficulties. Typically, patients complained of seeing people or obstacles "too late", bumping into them, and "getting lost" in busy places, supermarkets, or at "overcrowded" parties. All patients with increased scanning times, and also some with scanning times in the range of normal control subjects, reported such difficulties. In familiar environments, the majority of patients with unilateral field disorders reported much fewer problems. In contrast, patients with bilateral field defects also experienced some difficulties in familiar surroundings. Patients with left- and right-sided hemianopia complained of similar difficulties, while in the group of patients with quadranopia, especially patients with lower quadranopia, reported difficulties. Only 2 out of 14 patients with upper quadranopia reported that their vision is "far too slow", compared to 5 out of 7 patients with lower quadranopia. Thus, lower quadranopia seems to be more often associated with difficulties in everyday life than is upper quadranopia. This is in line with the notion that inferior areas of the visual field are most important for mobility (Lovie-Kitchin, Mainstone, Robinson, & Brown, 1990). Patients with hemiamblyopia reported fewer difficulties than did patients with hemianopia. Interestingly, among the 27 cases with homonymous amblyopia we found no subject who was unaware of the field disorder or attributed the visual problem to external factors. In contrast, 17 patients (32%) with left-sided and 12 (32%) with right-sided hemianopia, 5 patients (24%) with quadranopia, and 5 (out of 7) patients with bilateral hemianopia were unaware of their field loss. Furthermore, 7 patients (13%) with left-sided and 9 patients (24%) with right-sided hemianopia, and 3 patients (14%) with quadranopia attributed their visual difficulties to external factors. Such factors were, for example, changes in the (familiar) environment, inappropriate location of objects (e.g. chairs, plants, or street-lamps), "ill-mannered" people who either do not give way (when coming along on the patient's affected side) or frighten others (by reaching over from the affected side). The majority of cases in each subgroup (between 30% and 40%) reported "bad vision" without being able to provide a sufficient explanation for the worsening of their vision. Interestingly, many patients (77%) eventually decided that they should go to an ophthalmologist for the prescription of (new) glasses; others (15%) complained of "bad light" in the testing room; the rest were helpless. In total, 73.8% of our patients were without full insight into their visual problems or the origin of these problems. These observations are in agreement with the report by Celesia, Brigell, and Vaphiades (1997) who found a similarly high (62%) incidence in a group of 32 patients with homonymous field loss.

Patients with uni- ($n = 5$) or bilateral ($n = 5$) paracentral scotoma complained much less about "slow vision"; only two patients with bilateral paracentral scotoma reported that they often found it quite time-consuming to search for items lying on their desk, or to manage a dinner, especially when many different dishes were on the table. None of these patients reported particular difficulties in finding their way even in unfamiliar environments. However, all patients reported "strange" visual experiences; for example, that people or cars "suddenly" disappear and after a while reappear as fast as they had disappeared, but now much nearer and bigger, sometimes much too close so that they got a fright. The two patients with bilateral upper quadranopia reported some difficulties avoiding obstacles above them, and that sometimes it took them longer to get a complete view over their visual surroundings. However, they both found it "somehow exciting that the world is sharply cut in an upper and a lower half when I am looking straight ahead and then move my gaze upwards". In contrast, the two patients with bilateral lower quadranopia complained of being severely handicapped because they could not avoid (in time) obstacles lying on the floor. For example, they felt frightened because they did not notice dogs or small children until they barked or cried, respectively. Vision appeared very much slowed down to them, and they often got lost even in familiar environments. Interestingly, patients with paracentral scotoma as well as with bilateral upper or lower quadranopia were aware of their visual problems, and also correctly attributed these difficulties to their brain injury.

When evaluating these subjective reports, it is, of course, important to consider that patients may have compared their actual experience in these situations with experiences they had before suffering from brain injury. A patient who after brain injury shows a scanning performance within the range of age-matched control subjects may nevertheless complain of being impaired because the earlier (premorbid) performance may have been much better, and her or his behaviour in a particular situation may have been much more efficient. Patients therefore had to be asked very carefully about possible behavioural consequences of their field defect. In our group, only a small minority related the visual disability to their field loss; the others explained their difficulties either as a result of their "bad vision", or as caused by external factors. When asked what they themselves believe they should do to overcome their difficulties, only a few answered that they should "look more carefully". The majority assumed that new glasses would be adequate to improve their vision. Patients who may have had access to their field defect, either because they could detect visual stimuli in the affected field region (in cases with amblyopia), or because the incompleteness of perception can be directly experienced (in cases of paracentral scotoma), usually attributed their visual difficulties to the field defect. In conclusion, patients with homonymous visual field disorders are usually inaccurate in reporting their visual disabilities. The quality of their reports, however, can be considerably improved if they are confronted with items that are based on the behavioural effects of their visual deficit. Using a questionnaire for the assessment of visual disabilities in a group of 224 cases, we (Kerkhoff, Schaub, & Zihl, 1990) found that about 80% of subjects complained of difficulties in everyday life. Not noticing objects and bumping into them, losing one's way, not finding objects on a table, in a room or in a supermarket, and having difficulties to use public transportation were the items that received the highest ratings (Kerkhoff, Münssinger, & Meier, 1994).

In conclusion, the majority of patients with homonymous visual field disorders reported difficulties in everyday life; these claims are substantiated by eye movement recordings during the scanning of a visual display. However, the presence and severity of a homonymous field loss cannot sufficiently explain the observed impairment in oculomotor scanning. It appears that an additional factor is crucial for impaired oculomotor scanning, namely injury to occipitoparietal cortical areas or the posterior thalamus (Zihl, 1995b; see also p. 59).

RECOVERY FROM SCOTOMA BY SYSTEMATIC TRAINING

Experiments in primates with visual field defects after experimental striate cortex lesions have shown that systematic practice with detection and localisation of light stimuli resulted in a shrinkage of the scotoma (Cowey, 1967; Mohler & Wurtz, 1977). These results and observations of visual field enlargement in patients after regularly practice with various visual tasks (e.g. Pöppel, Brinkmann, von Cramon, & Singer, 1978) have stimulated researchers to find out whether patients with visual field loss after postchiasmatic injury could also possibly benefit from a similar type of systematic training. Patients received training in the detection of light stimuli presented at the border of the visual field ($n = 12$; Zihl & von Cramon, 1979) or in the saccadic localisation of light stimuli presented in the border zone and in the anopic field region ($n = 55$; Zihl, 1981; Zihl & von Cramon, 1985). Both procedures led to the recovery of visual field in some, but not all patients (Fig. 2.10). About 20% of patients did not show any significant change in field size; in 29 cases (43%) field enlargement did not exceed 5°. In single cases, however, considerable recovery was found; vision reappeared either in a large part of a hemifield or a quadrant. As in the experiments with monkeys reported by Mohler and Wurtz (1977), recovery was mainly observed in the field portion subjected to practice. In training-free intervals no further field enlargement was observed, indicating that recovery was linked to practice. Control experiments showed that field enlargement could not be explained by eccentric fixation, perimetric measurement variability, or the patient's or experimenter's expectation, as suggested by Balliett, Blood, and Bach-y-Rita (1985). Furthermore, these results have been essentially confirmed by other authors (Kasten & Sabel, 1995; Kerkhoff et al., 1992b; van der Wildt & Bergsma, 1997).

Based on the analysis of patients' brain lesions, we (Zihl & von Cramon, 1985) have speculated that visual field recovery can only be expected in cases with incomplete striate cortex injury, because no recovery was observed in patients with complete destruction of the striate cortex on the affected side. We have argued, therefore, that recovery from scotoma can be explained by a "reactivation" of reversibly injured cortical tissue. Attention may play a crucial role in processes of recovery by modulating the level of activation in striate cortex

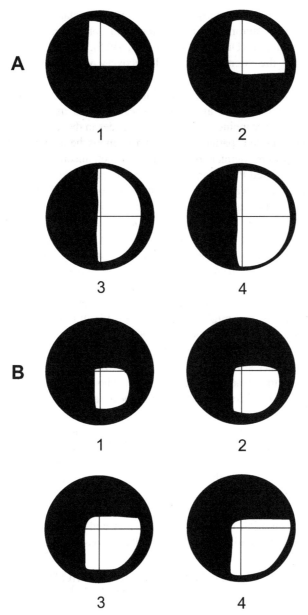

FIG. 2.10 Examples of visual field recovery (binocular testing condition) after systematic practice in two patients suffering from unilateral (A) and bilateral (B) occipital stroke. A: 42-year-old woman who had suffered right posterior cerebral infarction. Visual field was mapped 3 weeks (1), 6 weeks (2), 9 weeks (3), and 15 weeks (4) after stroke. B: 66-year-old man who had suffered bilateral posterior cerebral artery infarction. Visual fields were measured 3 weeks (1), 9 weeks (2), 15 weeks (3), and 23 weeks (4) after stroke. In both cases, treatment was carried out 9 weeks after brain injury.

neurons (Singer, 1979), thereby also modulating information processing and the interplay between "automatic" and "intentional" processes as well as between perception and action (Driver & Mattingley, 1995).

Interestingly, the extent of visual field recovery neither depended crucially on the age of the patient, nor on the "age" of the brain injury. The assumption that recovery of vision can only be expected in the case of reversible occipital injury is supported by Bosley et al. (1987). These authors used positron emission tomographic (PET) scanning to study serial changes in the local cerebral metabolic rate of glucose in five patients with homonymous hemianopia after occipital stroke. In two patients hemianopia disappeared spontaneously within 3–4 months, respectively; repeated PET scans showed improved striate cortex metabolism. In contrast, no recovery was found in the other patients, and PET scans showed no change in occipital metabolism. The authors concluded that the absence of metabolic activity indicates complete destruction of the striate cortex, and therefore irreversible visual field loss. Incomplete injury to the striate cortex, in contrast, is indicated by preserved although reduced metabolic activity in the affected brain region and might allow the preservation or recovery of the visual field.

Despite the positive results on partial recovery of the visual field after systematic practice, it soon became clear that these procedures are not useful for the majority of patients, and might in addition be difficult to implement in a clinical rehabilitation setting. Furthermore, as mentioned earlier, a valid and reliable measure that indicates whether a patient has a good or a poor prognosis for visual field recovery still does not exist. Any a priori selection of patients with a good prognosis for visual field recovery, i.e. who would be considered "qualified" or "appropriate" for this treatment, appears at least at present impossible. Furthermore, it may indeed be questioned whether patients can be expected to embark on a treatment procedure that consists of thousands of trials for the purpose of regaining a few degrees of visual field, if any (Gianutsos & Matheson, 1987).

Therefore, and because the number of patients with a sufficiently large visual field increase, which serves to reduce their visual handicap, is small, we decided to develop other methods of treatment. These methods aimed especially at an effective compensation of the visual field loss and were intended to be easily and successfully applied to as many patients as possible.

SUBSTITUTION BY OCULOMOTOR COMPENSATION

When considering methods of treatment for compensation, these methods should focus on the severity and frequency of the behavioural consequences of visual field disorders. Impairments in visual exploration and in reading represent the most common consequences; therefore, the main emphasis of treatment was on the acquisition of oculomotor strategies.

As described in the previous chapter, the majority of patients have difficulties developing an oculomotor strategy to compensate effectively for their visual field disorder. Oculomotor scanning patterns in these patients are characterised by hypometria, impaired visual orientation, and difficulties in glancing over the visual surroundings quickly enough to comprehend, for example, a scene as a whole. As a consequence, visual exploration is often unsystematic, irregular, and highly time-consuming. Interestingly, some patients show efficient spontaneous oculomotor adaptation to the field loss as soon as 2–3 weeks after the occurrence of brain injury (see Fig. 2.11 and Table 2.8). The majority of patients, however, may still exhibit insufficient compensation even several (i.e. 6–8) weeks post-injury. In a group of 60 patients with homonymous hemianopia only 40% developed oculomotor compensation strategies that were sufficiently effective for visual field substitution (Zihl, 1995b). In addition, since saccadic responses to acoustic targets may also be affected in these patients (Traccis et al., 1991), their difficulties may be exacerbated because the visual deficit cannot be compensated by the acoustic modality.

Based on the observations on patients' oculomotor scanning behaviour we developed a two-stage method of treatment (Zihl, 1988, 1990, 1995b). In the first phase, the use of large saccadic eye movements was practised to enlarge patients' field of search and to help them gain information where stimuli are located within a given spatial framework. In the second phase, patients learned to improve their scanning strategy, especially in regard to its spatial organisation. It should again be mentioned here that, according to the criteria proposed by Halligan et al. (1991), none of our patients exhibited signs of visual neglect.

Enlargement of saccade amplitudes

The main aim in enlarging saccadic eye movements in patients with homonymous visual field loss is to obtain a quick and almost complete view over the actual visual surroundings and thereby to extract information about its spatial structure and the distribution of visual stimuli, especially in the affected region. It is assumed that this overview enables the patient visually to guide the eye movements in a systematic and therefore efficient way. Scanning can then occur in a spatially and temporally coherent form, i.e. without loss of spatial orientation or temporal order of scanning, such that the patient can always know which part(s) of a scene or a stimulus array he or she has already inspected.

There are several possibilities of enlarging patients' saccades. Basically, a fixation stimulus (e.g. a red spot of light) and a target stimulus (a white light spot) can be used, with the distance between the two stimuli being variable within a range of 10–30° visual angle. The presentation time of the target should also be variable, typically between 5sec and 500msec. The background should be homogeneous and its structure should be uniform to prevent distraction. These prerequisites are best fulfilled by the Tübingen perimeter (Aulhorn &

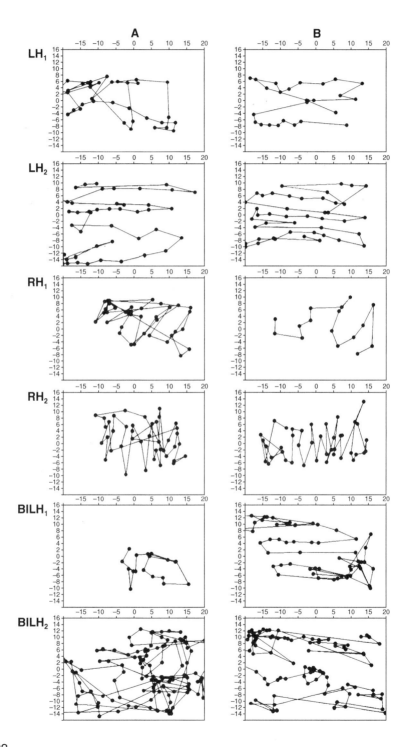

TABLE 2.8

Spontaneous oculomotor adaptation in 20 patients (12 males, 8 females; age = 48–68 years; $n = 5$ per group) with left- or right-sided hemianopia (field sparing < 5°) as assessed by recording eye movements in a dot counting task

Group	ST (sec) Mean (1SD)	FIX n (range)	FIXr (%) Mean (range)	A (°) Mean (1SD)
LH+/T1 (3–6)	24.8 (4.1)	48 (12)	28.4 (9–44)	5.6 (1.1)
LH+/T2 (2–6)	8.3 (1.1)	20 (5)	10.7 (6–13)	5.9 (0.9)
LH/T1 (3–8)	33.5 (7.7)	64 (11)	37.6 (14–59)	4.9 (0.6)
LH/T2 (4–9)	37.2 (6.7)	79 (27)	41.4 (11–54)	4.6 (1.1)
RH+/T1 (2–5)	28.4 (9.1)	55 (18)	34.5 (19–46)	5.8 (0.6)
RH+/T2 (4–11)	14.7 (6.5)	28 (8)	14.2 (6–23)	5.6 (1.1)
RH/T1 (3–6)	27.4 (8.4)	53 (21)	31.1 (14–43)	4.9 (0.5)
RH/T2 (3–9)	25.4 (7.6)	48 (24)	30.7 (19–41)	5.2 (0.8)
N	9.3 (0.8)	21 (4)	12.7 (6.2)	5.6 (0.7)

+: patients with successful adaptation. ST: search time; FIX: number of fixations; FIXr: repetition rates; A: saccadic amplitudes. T1: first testing (weeks since brain injury in brackets), T2: second testing (ranges of weeks since first testing in brackets); N: 30 normal age-matched control subjects for comparison.

Harms, 1972; Sloan, 1971), because target and background luminance conditions, target size, and presentation time can be exactly controlled. Furthermore, the perimeter allows the presentation of targets within the whole range of saccadic amplitudes. Such a large extent of the stimulus field is difficult to realise, if at all, by other means such as television screens or monitors. Using the Tübingen perimeter we presented targets along the horizontal axis in the affected hemifield, and along the main meridian in the affected visual field quadrant (see Fig. 2.12). Targets were shown in random order at least at three positions (mostly at 10°, 20°, and 30° eccentricity) along the corresponding field axis, with the minimal distance between target positions being 5°. The patient was comfortably seated with the head being maintained by a head and chin rest, and was informed that a light spot would appear for a limited time in the left or right hemifield. To enhance the control of attention, the corresponding axis and the closest and most distant positions of the target were shown to the patient at the beginning of the

FIG. 2.11   (opposite) Spontaneous oculomotor compensation in patients with left- (LH) and right-sided (RH) and with bilateral (BILH) hemianopia at time of first (A) and second (B) testing (4–6 weeks after A). Scanning times (in sec; A first value, B second): LH1 (3° sparing; 3 weeks post-injury): 10.5/10.0; LH2 (3°; 4 weeks): 20.1/21.7; RH1 (2°; 5 weeks): 10.1/10.8; RH2 (2°; 5 weeks): 18.7/19.7; BILH1 (9° central field sparing; 9 weeks): 18.5/25.6; BILH2 (11° central field sparing; 12 weeks): 43.5/53.6. LH and RH patients reported 20 dots; BILH1 reported 15 (A) and 18 dots (B), BILH2 12 (A) and 15 (B) dots. Further details as in Fig. 2.8.

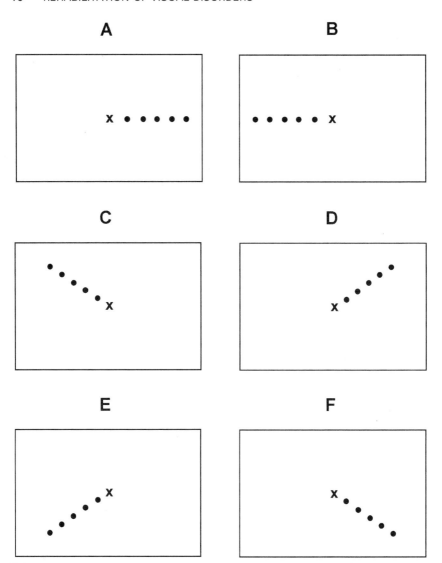

FIG. 2.12 Stimulus positions for practice with saccadic eye movements using the Tübingen peri-meter in patients with left-sided (A; left horizontal meridian) and right-sided (B; right horizontal meridian) hemianopia, and in patients with left upper (C; 135° meridian) and right upper (D; 45° meridian) quadranopia. In cases with lower quadranopia, targets were presented along the 225° meridian (left hemifield; E) and the 315° meridian (right hemifield; F).

sessions. The patient was then instructed to shift the eyes, without head move-ments, towards the indicated visual field region upon hearing an acoustic signal (evoked by the electromagnetic shutter at the perimeter). The saccadic eye move-ments should be executed as fast as possible and should be made as large as possible, so that even targets presented at more distant positions (e.g. at 30° eccentricity) could be seen in time. The rationale behind this procedure was to force the patient to shift the eyes in one large sweep from the fixation point to the position of the target. Patients were instructed rather to make a saccade larger (hypermetric) than the (expected) position of the target than to find the target by adding many small (hypometric) saccades. The patient was asked to press a response button after detection of the target. In order to achieve a detection rate of at least 60–70%, even at the beginning of the training phase, we usually started with a presentation time long enough to guarantee this level of performance. This turned out to be very helpful also for the patient's motivation and co-operation. In most patients the initial presentation time was 2sec; in patients with pronounced difficulties in using larger saccades, we used presentation times of up to 5sec. After a patient showed a detection rate of 95–100%, presentation time was systematically reduced to 500–300msec and practice continued until the patient showed a similarly high performance level in this condition. (This training procedure differed from that used in studies on "blindsight", where targets were presented for 100msec or less, and therefore could never be seen by the patient [Zihl, 1980]). Usually 5–6 sessions, each consisting of 90–120 target presentations (trials), were carried out. In the majority of patients (76%), 2–3 sessions were carried out per day; the rest participated in 1 session daily.

The effect of treatment was assessed by analysing horizontal saccades of 20° and 30° amplitude with respect to hypometria, by determining the extent of the field of view (field of gaze; Calabria et al., 1985; Courtney & Shou, 1985; Kerkhoff et al., 1994; Verriest et al., 1985; Zihl, 1990) using the Tübingen perimeter, and by recording the search time required to find 15 targets distributed in an array extending 52° horizontally and 45° vertically at a viewing distance of 140cm (see Fig. 2.13). The field of view was determined by asking the patient to leave the fixation point in the centre of the perimeter at the onset of the acoustic stimulus, and to search as quickly as possible for the light target, which was moved slowly at a speed of 1°/sec from the periphery towards the centre. Upon detecting the light target, the patient was requested to respond by pressing the buzzer key. Head movements were not allowed, so that the field of view would represent the useful field of gaze (Kerkhoff et al., 1994; Zihl & von Cramon, 1986b). All measurements were taken before and after treatment.

Tables 2.9A & B show the treatment procedure and the outcome of practice for two patients (P1, P2), both suffering from a complete left-sided hemianopia (field sparing = 1° in P1, and 1.5° in P2). Both patients showed pronounced saccadic hypometria, a severely restricted field of view, and a prolonged searching time, but differed with respect to their ability to use large saccadic eye movements. One patient (P1; Fig. 2.14) learned quite rapidly to use large saccades to the left (gain before = 0.86, after = 1.04), and showed an enlargement in the field of view by 26° and a striking reduction (before practice = 28.7sec; after practice = 17.2sec) in search time. The other patient (P2) required considerably ·

A

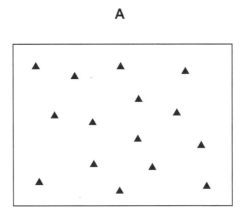

B

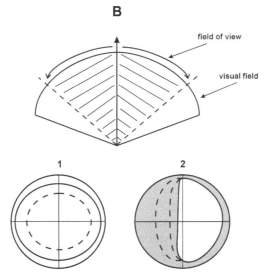

FIG. 2.13   Search test using a slide with 15 triangles as targets (A) and field of view (range of saccadic eye movements without head movements; B). The task in (A) was to count the targets while pointing at them with a light pointer. In (B), the extent of the visual field (outer lines) and of the field of view (hatched area within broken lines) are shown. B1: Normal visual field extent (continuous line) and extent of field of view (broken line); B2: example of left-sided hemianopia (grey area) and different extents of field of view (broken lines).

more practice, still exhibited saccadic hypometria after practice (gain before = 0.84, after = 0.92), achieved a smaller enlargement of the field of view (12°), and also a smaller reduction in search time (before practice = 28.1sec, after practice = 24.6sec). Table 2.10 shows the outcome in a group of 73 patients with left- or right-sided hemianopia. Similar to the two single cases, we found two

TABLE 2.9A
Enlargement of saccadic amplitudes:
Treatment procedure for two patients with left-sided
homonymous hemianopia (P1, P2)

Condition	Procedure
Centre → left	10°, 20°, 30° in random order
Presentation time	1sec or 0.5sec
P1	2 sessions/condition
P2	3 sessions/condition
Total number of trials	
P1	270
P2	450
Right ← centre → left	10°, 20°, 30° in random order
Presentation time	1sec or 0.5sec
P1	2 sessions/condition
P2	4 sessions/condition
Total number of trials	
P1	360
P2	720

TABLE 2.9B
Detection performance after practice (%).
Patient details as Table 2.9A

Condition	P1	P2
Centre → left		
1sec		
Session 1	78	64
Session 2	100	88
Session 3	–	98
0.5sec		
Session 4	84	72
Session 5	–	92
Centre → left or right		
1sec		
Session 1	88	78
Session 2	98	88
Session 3	–	92
Session 4	–	98
0.5sec		
Session 5	94	76
Session 6	98	86
Session 7	–	92
Session 8	–	96

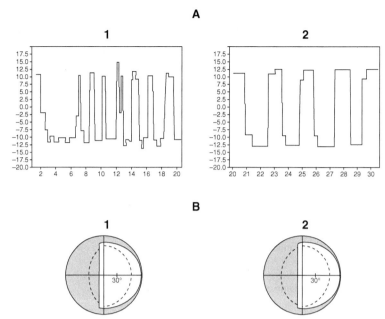

FIG. 2.14 Voluntary horizontal eye movements (A) and field of view (B) in a patient (P1 in Table 2.9) with left-sided hemianopia 6 weeks after occipital stroke before (1) and after (2) practice with large saccadic eye movements (420 trials). Bottom: left, top: right. x-axis: time period of recording (in sec); y-axis: horizontal amplitude (in degrees) of saccades (0 = centre). Dark area indicates lost field region. Note the pronounced hypometria and the small field of view before practice (1) compared with the moderate hypometria and considerably larger field of view after practice (2).

TABLE 2.10
Enlargement of saccadic amplitudes: Effect of practice on search time
(task in Fig. 2.13), field of view, and gain (for saccades into the
affected hemifield) in a group of patients with hemianopia

Patient group	Before M (1SD) M (range)	After M (1SD) M (range)	Sessions M (range)	Trials M (range)
Search time (sec)				
LH (n = 42)	31.6 (4.5)	22.9 (2.9)		
RH (n = 31)	32.0 (5.2)	23.1 (3.1)		
N (n = 25)	15.1 (2.1)			
Field of view (°)				
LH (n = 42)	9 (6–16)	30 (18–36)		
RH (n = 31)	11 (6–17)	31 (21–37)		
Gain				
LH (n = 42)	0.78 (0.62–1.10)	0.90 (0.76–1.06)		
RH (n = 31)	0.80 (0.71–1.08)	0.90 (0.78–1.08)		
Sessions and trials				
LH (n = 42)			4 (2–7)	450 (180–780)
RH (n = 31)			4 (2–8)	470 (210–880)

LH: left-sided, RH: right-sided hemianopia (field sparing < 10°); N: normal age-matched controls.

44

subgroups of patients: a smaller group ($n = 15$) with good improvement after 2–3 sessions, and a larger group ($n = 58$) with a smaller degree of improvement despite many more (4–8) training sessions. In addition, the latter group still showed a reduced saccadic gain, while gain was nearly normal in the first group. Interestingly, no differences were found between patients with left- and right-sided hemianopia. Mean time since brain injury (group 1: 8.4 weeks, range = 6–28 weeks; group 2: 8.6 weeks; range = 8–27 weeks) and mean age (group 1: 52.4 years; range = 28–74 years; group 2: 50.3 years; range = 27–72 years) were very similar in both groups. It appears highly unlikely, therefore, that these factors influenced the number of trials or the degree of improvement. As will be discussed in detail later (p. 59), the main underlying cause is the extent of brain injury.

All patients showed an improvement, although to a different degree, with the use of larger saccades after treatment not being restricted to the horizontal axis, which had been used for practice. Thus, the side towards which the shift of fixation (and, of course, attention) is directed appears to be crucial rather than the exact direction of the saccade.

The same training procedure was carried out in a group of 14 patients suffering from quadranopia. In this group, the use of large saccadic eye movements was practised along the main axis of the quadrant (see Fig. 2.12). As shown in Table 2.11, considerably fewer practice trials were required for the improvement

TABLE 2.11

Enlargement of saccadic amplitudes: Effect of practice on search time (task in Fig. 2.13), field of view (in degrees along the main axis in the anopic quadrant), and number of sessions/trials in 14 patients with quadranopia and in 8 patients with unilateral hemiamblyopia

Patient group	Before M (1SD)	After M (1SD)	Sessions M (range)	Trials M (range)
Search time (sec)				
UQ	21.8 (4.9)	17.9 (4.5)		
LQ	27.9 (4.7)	22.1 (4.3)		
HA	21.8 (3.2)	17.0 (2.8)		
N ($n = 25$)	15.1 (2.1)			
Field of view (°)				
UQ	11 (8–14)	24 (19–27)		
LQ	8 (6–12)	21 (16–24)		
HA	19 (14–26)	32 (27–39)		
Sessions and trials				
UQ			2 (2–3)	140 (90–170)
LQ			3 (2–4)	220 (120–280)
HA			2 (1–2)	90 (60–130)

UQ: unilateral upper quadranopia; LQ: unilateral lower quadranopia (field sparing < 10°); HA: unilateral hemiamblyopia (3 left-, 5 right-sided; sparing of form and colour vision < 10°); N: normal age-matched controls.

in this group than in the group of hemianopic patients, with patients with lower quadranopia on average requiring more trials than patients with upper quadranopia. Patients with upper quadranopia also showed less hypometria, larger fields of view, and shorter search times before treatment than patients with lower quadranopia; after treatment, these differences were no longer present.

In patients with homonymous hemiamblyopia ($n = 8$), the lowest number of trials (90 on average; see Table 2.11) was required to obtain a similar enlargement of saccadic eye movements as in the other groups. In comparison with patients suffering from hemianopia, patients with hemiamblyopia showed a smaller number of hypometric saccades, a fairly large field of view, and required less time to perform the search task before treatment. These observations might well be explained by the fact that these patients usually have no difficulties seeing a visual stimulus in their affected field region and can therefore use it to guide their saccades.

Statistical analysis (ANOVA) of the pre- and post-treatment data in patients with unilateral homonymous field defects ($n = 95$; Tables 2.10 and 2.11) revealed significant pre-post effects for search time ($F = 11.76$, and 323.57; $P < .001$) and field of view ($F = 19.53$ and 1835.9; $P < .001$) indicating that treatment has led to a highly significant reduction in search time and enlargement in the field of view. Significant pre- to post-treatment differences were found in each particular patient group (search time: $F > 58.77$; $P < .001$; field of view: $F > 148.08$; $P < .001$). No significant differences were found between groups concerning the enlargement of the field of view after practice. Furthermore, a significant negative correlation was found between search times and extent of the field of view before ($r = -.58$; $P < .001$) and after ($r = -.47$, $P < .001$) treatment, indicating that the larger the field of view, the higher the speed in visual search.

Patients with bilateral homonymous visual field disorders have difficulties using large eye movements that are directed to either hemifield. The treatment procedures and their assessment were identical to the ones described above, except that these patients required practice with large saccades to the left and to the right. We typically started with saccades to the left in the first part of the session, followed by practising saccades to the right. In the following session, the order was reversed. After achieving a sufficient level of performance, targets were presented in random order in the right or left hemifield. Tables 2.12A & B give examples of the order of practice and the corresponding results in two patients. Figure 2.15 shows horizontal saccades and the field of view in a patient with bilateral hemianopia before and after treatment. This patient did not only show increased saccadic accuracy after treatment, but also a considerable enlargement of his field of view. Patients with bilateral field disorders required considerably more practice than did patients with unilateral field disorders, with patients with bilateral hemiamblyopia showing the best outcome with the lowest number of trials. Even after a very intensive training period, patients with bilateral hemianopia and patients with bilateral lower quadranopia may not regain a full field of view and may still predominantly use hypometric saccades.

TABLE 2.12A
Enlargement of saccadic amplitudes: Treatment
procedure for a patient with bilateral homonymous
hemiamblyopia (BILHA) and a patient with
bilateral homonymous hemianopia (BILH)

Condition	Procedure
Left ← centre	10°, 20°, 30° in random order
Presentation times	1sec or 0.5sec
No. of sessions	
BILHA	2 sessions/condition
BILH	3 sessions/condition
No. of trials	
BILHA	360
BILH	540
Centre → right	10°, 20°, 30° in random order
Presentation time	1sec or 0.5sec
No. of sessions	
BILHA	2 sessions/condition
BILH	3 sessions/condition
No. of trials	
BILHA	360
BILH	540
Right ← centre → left	10°, 20°, 30° in random order
Presentation time	1sec or 0.5sec
No. of sessions	
BILHA	2 sessions/condition
BILH	3 sessions/condition
No. of trials	
BILHA	540
BILH	900

Nevertheless, an improvement in visual searching and an enlargement of the entire field of view was found after practice, in spite of the fact that practice was carried out along the horizontal or oblique field axes only (Table 2.13).

Although this phase of practice only consisted of enlargement of saccades directed towards the affected visual field region(s), about half of the patients reported less difficulties in their everyday lives when interviewed after practice (see Table 2.14). Thus, the use of larger eye movements has reduced the degree of impairment, especially in familiar environments. However, many patients (41.3%) still complained about difficulties with visual orientation and with the gaining of a "structured overview", as one patient put it, especially in unfamiliar or complex surroundings. We therefore decided to continue practice by using slides with large visual stimulus arrays and an increasing number of targets, and also added distractors in order to improve the spatial organisation of oculomotor scanning, and, as a result, visual orientation as well.

TABLE 2.12B
Detection performance after practice (%).
Patient details as Table 2.12A

Condition	BILHA	BILH
Left ← centre		
1sec		
Session 1	63	45
Session 2	86	68
Session 3	–	84
0.5sec		
Session 4	72	64
Session 5	88	76
Session 6	–	80
Centre → right		
1sec		
Session 1	76	78
Session 2	88	84
Session 3	–	88
0.5sec		
Session 4	78	66
Session 5	92	78
Session 6	–	80
Left ← centre → right		
1sec		
Session 1	76	54
Session 2	84	68
Session 3	92	72
Session 4	–	84
Session 5	–	78
0.5sec		
Session 6	84	66
Session 7	86	76
Session 8	94	82
Session 9	–	86
Session 10	–	84

Practice of visual search using slides

In this phase of practice patients were shown, at a distance of 140cm, stimulus arrays (52° × 45°) on slides, which contained between 5 and 20 numbers ranging in size between 0.5° and 3°, and distributed at random over the array (Fig. 2.16A). This stimulus condition is similar to the trail making test (Lezak, 1995), but numbers were not systematically arranged. Patients were asked to point to the individual numbers in an ascending order using a light pointer, and time was measured for error-free performance. The treatment was started with 5–10 items,

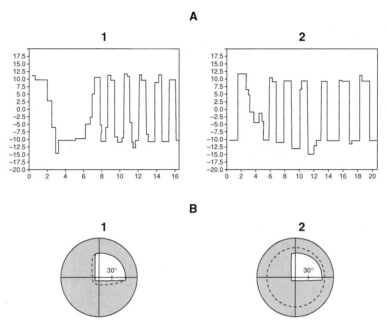

FIG. 2.15   Voluntary horizontal eye movements (A) and field of view (B) in a patient with bilateral homonymous field loss (patient BILH in Table 2.12) 8 weeks after bilateral occipital stroke before (1) and after (2) practice (1260 trials). Note the reduction of hypometria and the enlargement in the field of view after practice. Dark area indicates lost field region. For further details, see Fig. 2.14.

and the number of items was then increased in steps of five. After patients' search times were approximately within 90% of the time required by normal subjects, different shapes of the same size (triangles, squares, circles, stars) were used as stimuli (Fig. 2.16B). Patients were asked to search for the target items (e.g. triangles) among distractors (e.g. squares and circles), and after having found the target, to indicate it using a light pointer. Targets were randomly distributed among distractors. In the first sessions, 5–8 target items were shown among 10 distractors; in later sessions, the number of targets was increased stepwise up to 15 among at least 10 distractors. As in the first phase, the time for error-free searching performance was measured. Again, treatment was continued until patients' performance was at least 90% of normal subjects. Finally, in the last phase of this treatment, stimulus arrays were used with different forms (triangles, squares, stars) as distractors and letters (capitals) as target items (Fig. 2.16C). Each stimulus array contained 5–10 targets among 15–20 distractors, but set size (25 items in total) was kept constant. Between 10 and 15 blocks were carried out in one session, which consisted of 15–20 trials each. Patients were instructed to search for an individual target stimulus indicated by the

TABLE 2.13
Enlargement of saccadic amplitudes: Effect of practice on searching and field of
view (Fig. 2.13) in a group of 14 patients with bilateral homonymous field loss

Patient group	Before M (1SD; range)	After M (1SD; range)	Sessions M (range)	Trials M (range)
Search time (sec)				
BILH	45.9 (8.2)	34.2 (6.7)		
BILUQ	30.7 (28–32)	11.9 (23–24)		
BILLQ	37.0 (36–38)	26.2 (25–27)		
BILHA	31.8 (3.3)	23.8 (2.8)		
N (n = 25)	15.1 (2.1)			
Field of view (°)				
BILH (n = 5)	12.4 (4.6)	39.6 (6.7)		
BILUQ (n = 2)	07.0 (6–8)	19.5 (18–21)		
BILLQ (n = 2)	5.5 (5–6)	18.0 (17–19)		
BILHA (n = 5)	28.6 (3.0)	53.4 (3.6)		
Sessions and trials				
BILH (n = 5)			6 (4–8)	720 (520–920)
BILUQ (n = 2)			3 (3)	210 (110–260)
BILLQ (n = 2)			4 (3–4)	490 (390–510)
BILHA (n = 5)			4 (3–5)	470 (320–540)

BILH: patients with bilateral hemianopia; BILUQ, BILLQ: patients with bilateral upper or
lower quadranopia; BILHA: patients with bilateral amblyopia; N: normal age-matched controls.
For n < 5, the ranges are given. Field of view: mean diameter in patients with bilateral hemianopia
or amblyopia. For further details, see Table 2.11.

TABLE 2.14
Report of patients with homonymous visual field loss about difficulties
in their everyday life in unfamiliar surroundings before and after
enlargement of saccadic eye movements

	LH (n = 42)		RH (n = 31)		Q (n = 14)	
	Before	After	Before	After	Before	After
Vision "too slow"	86	57	77	51	43	36*
Bumping against obstacles	55	17	54	16	28	21*
"Getting lost"	48	14	22	3	14	7*

LH: patients with left-sided hemianopia; RH: patients with right-sided hemianopia; Q: patients
with quadranopia. Reports refer mainly to unfamiliar surroundings (cf. Table 2.7). Numbers refer
to percentages of patients. *Patients with lower quadranopia.

experimenter (e.g. the letter "T"), with targets varying between trials. Treatment
was finished after a patient showed a search speed which was at least 90% found
in the same condition in a group of normal control subjects. Search performance
was assessed before and after practice using parallel versions of two different

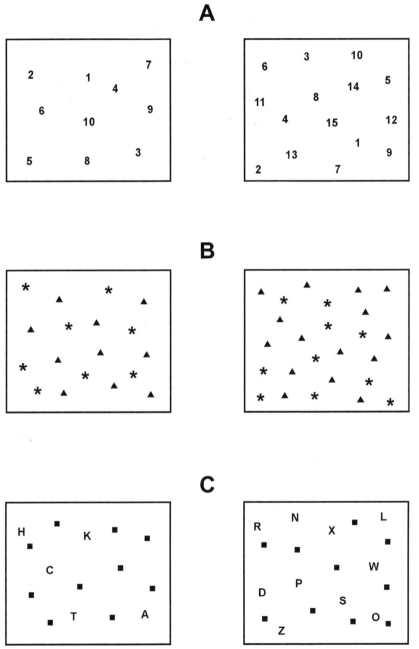

FIG. 2.16 Training slides for practice with visual scanning using different stimuli and stimulus densities on slides. A: numbers; B: triangles (targets) among stars (distractors); C: letters (targets) among forms (distractors).

stimulus arrays (Fig. 2.17). Patients were asked to search for numbers in an ascending order (1–20) which were arranged randomly over the array. The second array contained 20 diamonds as targets embedded in 22 distractors (circles, crosses). In both cases, subjects used a light pointer to indicate the location of the particular targets. In Tables 2.15 and 2.16 the results for the various groups of patients with homonymous field defects are shown. Improved scanning performance was found in every patient group; however, about one third (27%) of patients with unilateral and all patients with bilateral field loss still required more time than did normal subjects.

A

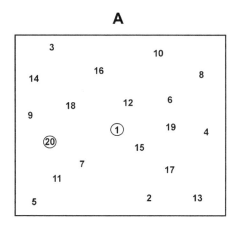

B

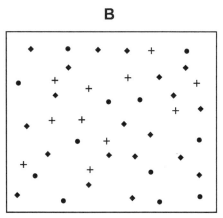

FIG. 2.17   Stimulus arrays to assess visual scanning performance. A: connecting of numbers from 1–20 in ascending order; B: counting of targets (diamonds; $n = 20$) among distractors (circles, crosses). Subjects were asked to point at each target (A: numbers; B: diamonds).

TABLE 2.15

Search performance (in seconds; $n = 10$ per condition) in two visual tasks (A: connection of numbers from 1–20; B: searching for 20 diamonds among 42 items) in 100 patients with unilateral field loss before and after practice with visual scanning on slides

Group	A Before M (1SD)	A After M (1SD)	B Before M (1SD)	B After M (1SD)	S n (range)
LHa ($n = 31$)	48.8 (4.8)	39.3 (3.4)	15.9 (2.8)	13.6 (1.8)	4 (3–5)
LHb ($n = 11$)	57.3 (4.8)	48.2 (5.4)	18.7 (2.1)	15.9 (1.9)	8 (6–9)
RHa ($n = 21$)	47.3 (5.1)	40.4 (2.5)	16.2 (2.1)	13.4 (1.8)	5 (4–6)
RHb ($n = 10$)	53.3 (5.2)	48.1 (3.6)	18.4 (1.3)	15.7 (1.1)	9 (6–10)
Qa ($n = 11$)	45.8 (2.5)	39.7 (2.3)	15.1 (0.3)	13.1 (0.4)	3 (3–4)
Qb ($n = 3$)	49.8 (3.8)	43.9 (3.2)	16.7 (1.6)	14.8 (0.9)	5 (5–6)
HAa ($n = 5$)	46.3 (2.2)	39.6 (1.1)	14.9 (0.2)	13.7 (0.3)	3 (3–4)
HAb ($n = 3$)	51.5	44.8	16.4	14.4	5 (4–6)
PCS ($n = 5$)	43.7 (1.3)	40.2 (1.1)	15.1 (0.3)	13.5 (0.4)	3 (2–4)
N ($n = 25$)	38.7 (3.6)		13.2 (1.3)		

LH: patients with left-sided hemianopia ($n = 42$); RH: with right-sided hemianopia ($n = 31$); Q: with quadranopia ($n = 14$); HA: unilateral hemiamblyopia ($n = 8$); PCS: patients with unilateral paracentral scotoma ($n = 5$). a: patients with good improvement, b: patients with poor improvement (performance 2 SD lower than normal subjects). S: number of sessions. N: mean search time in a group of age-matched normal control subjects for comparison.

TABLE 2.16

Search performance (in seconds; $n = 10$ per condition) in two visual tasks (A: connection of numbers from 1–20; B: searching for 20 diamonds among 42 items) in 19 patients with bilateral field loss before and after practice with visual scanning on slides

Group	A Before M (1SD)	A After M (1SD)	B Before M (1SD)	B After M (1SD)	S n (range)
BILH ($n = 5$)	64.2 (6.9)	50.3 (4.5)	28.9 (3.5)	16.8 (3.2)	11 (8–13)
BILHA ($n = 5$)	49.4 (4.3)	44.2 (2.8)	16.7 (2.1)	14.4 (1.9)	7 (4–10)
BILQ ($n = 4$)	54.7	45.6	15.9	14.6	5 (3–7)
BILPCS ($n = 5$)	49.2 (2.1)	36.8 (2.4)	17.8 (0.6)	15.2 (0.4)	6 (4–7)
N ($n = 25$)	38.7 (3.6)		13.2 (1.3)		

BILH: patients with bilateral hemianopia; BILHA: with bilateral hemiamblyopia; BILQ: with bilateral (upper and lower) quadranopia; BILPCS: with bilateral paracentral scotomata. S: number of sessions. N: mean search time in a group of age-matched normal control subjects for comparison.

Statistical analysis of data using ANOVA again revealed significant treatment effects for both search time ($F = 413.69$; $P < .001$) and field of view ($F = 571.85$; $P < .001$). This also holds true for each particular group (search time: smallest $F > 43.48$; $P < .001$; field of view: $F > 82.04$; $P < .001$). Again, a significant negative correlation was found between the extent of the field of view and the search time before ($r = -.58$; $P < .001$) and after ($r = -.67$; $P < .001$) practice. This supports the view that patients with a smaller field of view required more time to search for the stimuli while patients with a larger field of view required less time both before and after treatment.

In addition to the assessment of search performance and field of view, we recorded eye movements before and after practice of visual scanning. A pattern of randomly distributed dots was used as the stimulus array (see Fig. 2.6B). Figures 2.18 and 2.19 show the eye movements of individual subjects with left-sided, right-sided or bilateral hemianopia. After practice, an improvement in the scanning pattern is evident in all three subjects. Figure 2.20 and Tables 2.17 and 2.18 summarise the outcome of a larger patient group ($n = 58$) suffering from uni- or bilateral homonymous field disorders. Compared to the before-treatment performance, all patients showed a marked reduction in scanning time, length of scan path, number of fixations and especially of repetition of fixations, and also in the mean duration of fixations. In addition, mean saccadic amplitudes were larger after treatment.

Statistical analysis (ANOVA) of eye movement parameters revealed significant ($P < .001$) pre-post differences for scanning time ($F = 181.14$), fixations ($F = 214.90$), repetition of fixations ($F = 217.46$), fixation durations ($F = 400.01$), and saccadic amplitudes ($F = 174.85$). Significant ($P < .001$) differences between pre- and post-treatment results were also found in each subgroup (search time: $F > 62.03$; fixations: $F > 49.39$; fixation repetitions: $F > 73.84$; fixation durations: $F > 101.77$; saccadic amplitudes: $F > 38.64$). Thus, all patient groups showed significantly improved scanning parameters after practice indicating that the oculomotor scanning patterns were indeed considerably improved by the treatment strategy adopted.

Despite the significant improvements in all patient groups, not all subjects reached the level of "normal" performance. If the highest time value (13sec) of 30 normal control subjects is used as a reference, then 30 (52%) patients still performed below this level. In the groups with hemianopia or quadranopia, half of the patients required more time, while in the group with hemiamblyopia only one patient did not perform normally. In contrast, three out of five patients with bilateral paracentral scotoma, the two patients with bilateral lower quadranopia, all five patients with bilateral hemianopia, and four out of five patients with bilateral hemiamblyopia did not reach normal scanning performance.

Summarising these observations, one can conclude that patients' visual search performance and oculomotor scanning patterns were more efficient after practice in terms of their spatiotemporal parameters, resulting in a more rapid and accurate

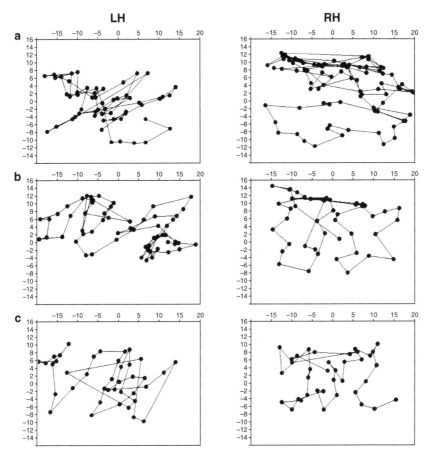

FIG. 2.18 Oculomotor scanning patterns during the scanning of a dot pattern (see Fig. 2.6B) in patients with left-sided (LH; field sparing = 2°) and with right-sided (RH; field sparing = 1.5°) homonymous hemianopia at time of first testing (a; 7 and 8 weeks post-injury), before (b; 4 weeks later) and after (c) practice with visual scanning on slides (LH: 840 trials; RH: 880 trials). x-axis: horizontal extension of stimulus array (in degrees; 0 = centre, negative values left, positive values right), y-axis: vertical extension (0 = centre, negative values down, positive values up). Dots indicate fixation locations. Both patients reported correctly 20 dots in all testing occasions. Scanning times (in sec): LH: a: 27.4, b: 25.7, c: 16.0; RH: a: 30.1, b: 26.1, c: 13.8. For comparison, mean scanning time in a group of 30 age-matched normal control subjects was 9.3 sec (range = 6.2–12.8).

overview and also in a more systematic organisation of the scanpath. As a consequence, patients were expected to be more efficient in compensating for their field loss and to experience less difficulties in everyday life conditions. This was indeed the case, at least for most of the patients who performed in the normal range after treatment. As Table 2.19 shows, the majority of patients no longer complained that their vision was "too slow" after treatment. Furthermore,

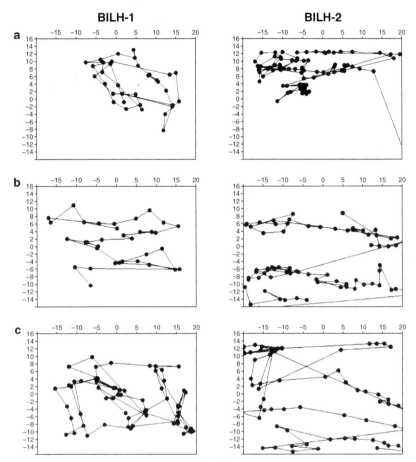

FIG. 2.19 Oculomotor scanning patterns during the scanning of a dot pattern (see Fig. 2.6B) in two patients with bilateral homonymous hemianopia (BILH1: central field sparing = 12°; BILH2: central field sparing = 14°) at time of first testing (a) (BILH1: 9 weeks, BILH2: 11 weeks post-injury), before (b; 5 weeks later) and after practice (c) with visual scanning on slides (BILH1: 2210 trials; BILH2: 2280 trials). Patient BILH1 reported 7 out of 20 dots (a), 13 dots (b), and 17 dots after practice (c), while patient BILH2 reported 13 dots (a), 15 dots (b), and 18 dots (c) after practice. Scanning times (in sec): BILH: a: 19.9, b: 19.4, c: 27.1; BILH2: a: 61.4, b: 61.5, c: 43.6. For comparison, mean scanning time in a group of 30 age-matched normal control subjects was 9.3 sec (range = 6.2–12.8). Further details as in Fig. 2.18.

no patient with a unilateral field defect reported bumping into obstacles or people and only a few cases still complained of getting lost. In a familiar environment, nearly all patients reported that after treatment they could do everything they could before the stroke. In more unfamiliar environments, some patients, however, still experienced difficulties, especially regarding their visual orientation. Interestingly, all patients were now fully aware of their field loss and its consequences

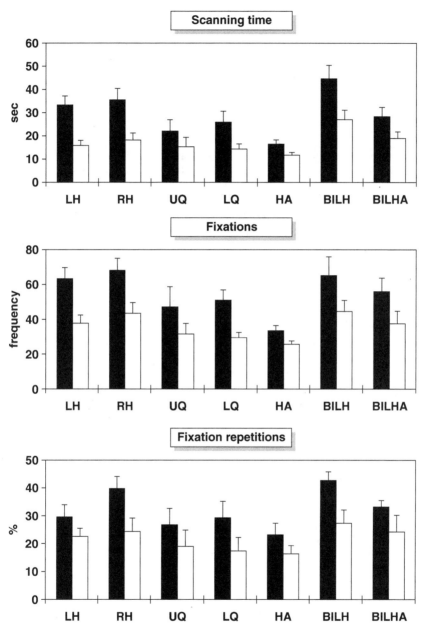

FIG. 2.20 Scanning time, number of fixations, and rate of fixation repetitions in patients with left-sided (LH; $n = 17$) or right-sided (RH; $n = 16$) hemianopia; upper (UQ; $n = 5$) or lower (LQ; $n = 5$) quadranopia; hemiamblyopia (HA; $n = 5$); bilateral hemianopia (BILH; $n = 5$); or bilateral hemiamblyopia (BILHA; $n = 5$) before (dark bars) and after (white bars) practice with visual scanning on slides. Note decrease in scanning times, number of fixations, and rates of fixation repetition in each patient group.

TABLE 2.17
Fixation durations and saccadic amplitudes during oculomotor scanning of a dot
pattern (see Fig. 2.6) before and after practice with visual scanning on slides in
48 patients with unilateral field loss

	FD (sec)		A (°)	
Group	Before M (1SD)	After M (1SD)	Before M (1SD)	After M (1SD)
LH (n = 17)	0.29 (0.05)	0.26 (0.03)	4.5 (0.9)	5.1 (0.9)
RH (n = 16)	0.31 (0.10)	0.28 (0.06)	4.8 (0.9)	5.1 (1.1)
UQ (n = 5)	0.32 (0.09)	0.27 (0.07)	5.4 (0.8)	5.4 (0.4)
LQ (n = 5)	0.30 (0.05)	0.26 (0.04)	5.2 (1.3)	5.4 (0.3)
HA (n = 5)	0.28 (0.09)	0.24 (0.04)	4.5 (0.5)	5.6 (0.6)
N (n = 30)	0.27 (0.02)		5.6 (0.7)	

LH: patients with left-sided; RH: with right-sided hemianopia; UQ: with upper; LQ: with
lower quadranopia; HA: patients with hemiamblyopia; N: the corresponding values for a group
of normal subjects are shown for comparison.

TABLE 2.18
Oculomotor scanning (dot counting task) before and after practice with
visual scanning on slides in 19 patients with bilateral visual field loss:
Fixation durations (FD) and saccadic amplitudes (A)

	FD (sec)		A (°)	
Group	Before M (1SD)	After M (1SD)	Before M (1SD)	After M (1SD)
BILH (n = 5)	0.35 (0.06)	0.28 (0.03)	4.1 (0.5)	5.4 (0.5)
BILHA (n = 5)	0.28 (0.05)	0.25 (0.04)	4.8 (0.5)	5.2 (0.9)
BILQ (n = 4)	0.31	0.24	5.1	5.5
BILPCS (n = 5)	0.27 (0.01)	0.26 (0.03)	5.1 (1.1)	5.8 (1.2)

BILH: bilateral hemianopia; BILHA: bilateral hemiamblyopia; BILQ: bilateral (upper or
lower) quadranopia; BILPCS: bilateral paracentral scotomata. For corresponding values in normal
control subjects, see Table 2.17.

TABLE 2.19
Report of 43 patients with unilateral homonymous visual field loss about
difficulties in their everyday life in unfamiliar surroundings before and
after practice with visual scanning on slides

	LH (n = 17)		RH (n = 16)		Q (n = 10)	
	Before n	After n	Before n	After n	Before n	After n
Vision "too slow"	17	4	16	5	10	3*
Bumping against obstacles	14	0	12	1	7	1*
"Getting lost"	11	0	8	0	4	1*

LH: patients with left-sided hemianopia; RH: patients with right-sided hemianopia; Q: patients
with quadranopia. Reports refer mainly to unfamiliar surroundings (cf. Table 2.7). *patients with
lower quadranopia.

in everyday life activities. It appears, therefore, that the combination of enlarging saccadic eye movements and improving oculomotor scanning and thereby also visual orientation resulted in a considerable decrease of the visual handicap. However, as mentioned above, more than one third (38%) of patients still reported some difficulties. These difficulties occurred mainly in situations where visual orientation is of absolute importance, for example when shopping in supermarkets and finding the way in crowded places.

Thus, it can be concluded that patients with homonymous uni- or bilateral visual field defects can benefit from a treatment specifically devoted to the learning of oculomotor compensation strategies to substitute their lost or affected visual field regions. Using similar methods, Pommerenke and Markowitsch (1989) and Kerkhoff et al. (1994) reported comparable improvements in their patients.

As patients' reports indicate, there is a clear treatment effect on the reduction of the visual handicap in everyday life. Of course, in order to present more objective data on this issue, a systematic observation of patients' behaviour in standardised conditions of everyday life activities would be required. On the other hand, the fact that all patients in our study were already fully aware of their difficulties before treatment suggests that their reports on their visual handicap were adequate and sufficiently reliable. Certainly, one has to take into account each patient's self-assessment of the ability to gain a quick and reliable view over the visual surroundings, to get one's bearings and to find one's way without major difficulties. There is no doubt that subjects can differ considerably with respect to these visual abilities, and thus subjects may have already been different before the stroke. These individual differences between patients might also help to explain why some patients were very much surprised by their own observation that after treatment they "can see at least as well as before or even better", while others agreed they had improved, but were still concerned that they had not reached the level of performance they had before brain injury. In explaining the degree of improvement and the beneficial effects on everyday life activities, it therefore appears necessary to take into account the individual patient's self-assessment and to give appropriate and helpful advice concerning any special conditions of the individual's everyday life.

A further comment appears necessary regarding the group of patients who showed clear improvement after treatment and were also able to transfer their compensation strategies to everyday life, but still exhibited some impairment. In searching for an explanation we found that these patients also suffered from injury to occipitoparietal structures, the posterior thalamus, or both. The posterior thalamus and its reciprocal connections with cortical regions in the occipital, parietal, and frontal lobes, and limbic neocortex are assumed to be part of a cortical–subcortical network subserving attention and saccadic movements, intentionally guided as well as externally triggered, involved in visual information processing (Corbetta et al., 1993; Kustov & Robinson, 1996; Mesulam, 1981;

Petersen, Robinson, & Morris, 1987; Pierrot-Deseilligny et al., 1995; Robinson, 1993; Robinson & Petersen, 1992; Selemon & Goldman-Rakic, 1988). Furthermore, fibre pathways connecting occipital, parietal, temporal, and frontal cortical areas coursing in the occipital white matter (Morel & Bullier, 1990; Rockland & Pandya, 1981; Seltzer & Pandya, 1984), might also have been injured in these patients, thus interrupting connections between these areas as well. It is therefore not surprising that patients with additional injury to these structures have more difficulties with the visual spatial guidance of their attention and their eye movements in addition to the impairments caused by the visual field loss *per se* (Zihl, 1995b). Injury to the thalamus or to occipitoparietal structures is not uncommon in posterior stroke. For example, Goto et al. (1979) found involvement of these structures in 17 (44.7%) out of 38 patients with posterior cerebral artery occlusion. Thus, in these patients we are dealing with a "homonymous visual field loss plus visual disorientation syndrome". It is important to note that this combined visual disorder is not only present in patients with right-sided or bilateral brain injury but also in cases with left-sided posterior brain injury, indicating that visual orientation depends crucially on the functional integrity and interaction of both hemispheres.

Despite the improvements observed so far by means of enlarging saccadic eye movements and improving visual searching and scanning, we searched for a more flexible and thus more effective type of practice especially focused on visual scanning and visual orientation. A computer-based program allows more individual specifications with respect to the number, type, and presentation time of visual stimuli and the level of difficulty of the task involved. Since the searching for and scanning of targets has proved successful in acquiring an effective compensation strategy, we decided to use the visual search paradigm as the principal type of task. This paradigm was developed to investigate modes of processing as a function of the number and type of visual stimuli. The typical task of a subject is to search for a target embedded in a set of non-targets (distractors). Based on the characteristics of the target and distractor stimuli used (for example, colour, size, or form), two main types of processing can be distinguished: The so-called parallel or automatic processing mode, where the search time does not increase when the number of distractors is increased, and the so-called serial processing mode, where searching time increases with increasing set size (for a more detailed description and theoretical discussion of the visual search paradigm in neuropsychology, see Humphreys & Riddoch, 1994, and Robertson, 1992). There is evidence that this visual task not only comprises the processing of visual stimuli, but also visual-spatial attention (Chelazzi, Miller, Duncan, & Desimone, 1993). We hypothesised that the improvement in the interaction between visual search and spatial shift of attention would be a powerful tool for the improvement of patients' oculomotor compensation strategy, since selective attention is known to enhance the capacity to process information at lower and higher visual cortical levels (e.g. Cowey, 1994; Singer, 1979).

Practice of visual search using the search paradigm

Visual search was tested and practised using a PC-based system with a 17-inch high-resolution monitor. The subject sat at a distance of 60cm in front of the screen. A specially developed software program was responsible for the generation and presentation of the stimuli as well as for the recording of subjects' responses. The schematic drawing in Fig. 2.21 shows the stimulus conditions and the temporal course of two trials. The subject was instructed to fixate the blue cross in the centre of the monitor and to search, after the disappearance of the cross, for a single target known to the subject (e.g. a red E), which was embedded among distractors (e.g. green Fs). When the target was present on the monitor, the subject was to press the left mouse button ("target-button"), while the right button was to be pressed when no target was present. For treatment we used target/distractor combinations which included "parallel", "mixed", and "serial" search conditions (Table 2.20). Each stimulus condition consisted of 15 items (set size), either of one target and 14 distractors, or of 15 distractors. Practice in individual patients was always started with the easiest ("parallel") condition, followed by the "mixed" condition, and finally the "serial" condition. The subjects were instructed to search as carefully as possible for the target, but at the same time also as quickly as possible, i.e. they should not respond until they were sure that a target was present or absent. Typically 20 trials were carried out in one block and each practice session consisted of 10–15 blocks. Thus one session consisted of 200–300 trials and lasted, breaks included, 30–45min, depending on the response times of a patient. The change from "parallel" to "mixed" and from "mixed" to "serial" conditions was not carried out before a patient showed clear improvement and searched at a stable level of performance in a particular task condition.

In using the visual search paradigm as an alternative treatment procedure for patients with homonymous visual field defects, we were not only interested to find out whether this procedure might be a valuable method of practice, but also whether we could find a transfer from the smaller (the monitor) to a larger field of search (a slide; see Fig. 2.17B, p. 52). This transfer appears to be crucial considering the fact that patients should gain compensatory strategies for everyday life, where an overview is often required for quite large surroundings. To assess the improvement made through this method of practice, we used our standard visual search condition (target: E, distractor: F; see Fig. 2.21) before and after practice. In addition, we recorded eye movements during the scanning of a dot pattern (see Fig. 2.6B), and measured the field of view.

Two groups of patients were treated with the visual search method: 9 patients with left-sided, and 8 patients with right-sided hemianopia (for clinical details, see Table 2.21). Table 2.22 shows the procedure of treatment for two individual patients and the corresponding results. After about 400 trials in the "parallel"

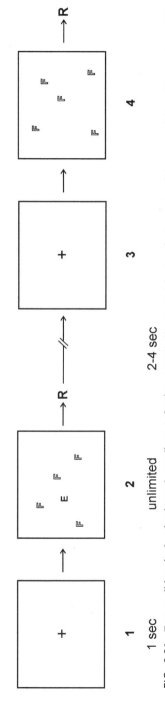

FIG. 2.21 Test conditions in the visual search paradigm. A fixation cross (1, 3) appeared for 1sec in the centre of the screen, followed by a pattern of F's (distractors) and one E (target) (2), or no target at all (4). Presentation time was unlimited; the next presentation was started 2–4sec after subject's response (R).

TABLE 2.20

Target/distractor conditions used in the treatment of patients with homonymous visual field loss. Examples for "parallel", "mixed", and "serial" searching conditions. A total of 15 items were used per condition, with 7–8 targets

"Parallel" (Target–Distractor)	"Mixed" (Target–Distractor)	"Serial" (Target–Distractor)
I–O	T–S	C–D
O–T	A–L	O–G
N–O	S–O	I–L
S–A	L–A	R–K
H–C	S–C	T–I
A–U	O–U	G–C
V–G	C–O	V–A
U–P	D–O	B–D

TABLE 2.21

Clinical details of 17 patients (2 females, 15 males) with hemianopia after occipital stroke participating in the practice with visual search

Group	Age (years) M (range)	T (weeks) M (range)	VFSP (°) M (range)
LH (n = 9)	54 (23–79)	16 (9–28)	2.7 (1–4)
RH (n = 8)	51 (40–65)	14 (8–22)	2.9 (1–4)

LH: patients with left-; RH: with right-sided hemianopia.
T: time since brain injury; VFSP: visual field sparing.

search condition, both hemianopic patients showed a clear reduction in search time, and no more omissions. A similar outcome was obtained in the "mixed" and in the "serial" searching conditions, but more trials were required to reach a stable level of improvement. Figure 2.22 shows the performance in the visual search task before and after treatment. Interestingly, before treatment 13 patients were unable to search in parallel even in typical "parallel" search conditions; after treatment 7 patients still showed a serial searching behaviour in "parallel" conditions. In spite of this, search times were considerably reduced after treatment in all groups. Table 2.23 summarises the pre- to post-treatment data on the two groups of patients concerning searching times (task shown in Fig. 2.17B) and extent of the field of view. There is a clear enlargement of the field of search and a considerable decrease in the time required to find the targets.

Statistical analysis (ANOVA) of data revealed significant treatment effects for search time ($F = 455.49$; $P < .001$) and field of view ($F = 360.54$; $P < .001$). The significant differences were observed in each subgroup for both search time ($F > 93.34$; $P < .001$) and field of view ($F > 100.80$; $P < .001$). No significant

TABLE 2.22
Practice with visual search: Plans of treatment
and outcome in two patients with hemianopia

	First session	Last session
LH		
"Parallel" condition (after 390 trials)		
Time (msec)	1040	710
Errors	0/3	0/0
"Mixed" condition (after 615 trials)		
Time (msec)	1920	870
Errors	0/4	0/1
"Serial" condition (after 435 trials)		
Time (msec)	1980	1380
Errors	0/3	0/1
RH		
"Parallel" condition (after 435 trials)		
Time (msec)	990	770
Errors (M/1SD)	1/2	0/0
"Mixed" condition (after 450 trials)		
Time (msec)	1540	810
Errors (M/1SD)	0/2	0/1
"Serial" condition (after 225 trials)		
Time (msec)	1610	1180
Errors (M/1SD)	0/4	1/1
Normal subjects		
"Parallel" condition		
Time (msec)	520 (47.3)	
Total errors (M/1SD)	0/1	
"Mixed" condition		
Time (msec)	655 (58.4)	
Total errors (M/1SD)	1/1	
"Serial" condition		
Time (msec)	913 (90.5)	
Total errors (M/1SD)	1/2	

LH: male, 46 years; time since brain injury = 16 weeks; field sparing = $2°$, RH: male, 48 years; time since brain injury = 17 weeks; field sparing = $2°$. Search times for targets (mean and 1 SD; 20 trials) and errors (false negatives/false positives) in the first and in the last training session. For comparison, results of 10 normal subjects (20 trials per condition) are shown. Targets/distractors: "parallel" condition O/T; "mixed" condition C/O; "serial" condition G/C.

main group effect was found, indicating that left- and right-sided hemianopic patients did not differ significantly before and after practice with respect to search performance and field of view. In addition a significant negative correlation between search time and extent of the field of view was found before ($r = -.75$; $P < .001$) and after ($r = -.56$; $P < .05$) treatment, confirming the earlier

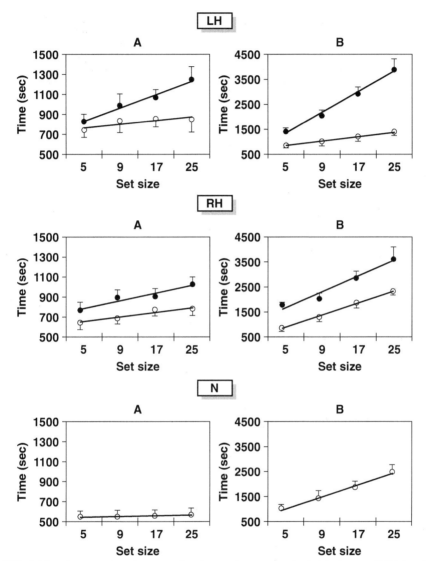

FIG. 2.22   Visual search performance (time in seconds; means and 1 SD) in the "parallel"(A) and "serial"(B) search conditions in patients with left-sided (LH; $n = 9$) and right-sided (RH; $n = 8$) hemianopia before (closed circles) and after (open circles) practice with visual search. Set size: number of items. Vertical bars: 1SD. Note the reduction in search time after practice of both groups in both conditions. For comparison, corresponding data of 10 age-matched normal subjects (N) are shown.

(pp. 46 and 54) found association between the extent of the field of view and the speed in visual search.

The improvement in visual search was paralleled by a marked change in the eye movement pattern during visual scanning, as Fig. 2.23 shows. The patients

TABLE 2.23
Effect of practice with visual search on performance in a search task
(Fig. 2.17B) and field of view in a group of patients with left-sided and
with right-sided hemianopia. See text for further details

Patient group	Before M (1SD)	After M (1SD)	Sessions M (range)	Trials M (range)
Search time (sec)				
LH (n = 9)	37.4 (6.2)	19.8 (5.8)		
RH (n = 8)	34.1 (8.3)	21.8 (7.8)		
N (n = 25)	13.2 (1.3)			
Field of view (°)				
LH (n = 9)	13.0 (3.7)	32.7 (4.6)		
RH (n = 8)	12.8 (5.7)	30.8 (4.4)		
Sessions and trials				
LH (n = 9)			6 (5–7)	1220 (990–1440)
RH (n = 8)			7 (5–8)	1330 (960–1520)

LH: left-sided hemianopia; RH: right-sided hemianopia, N: normal subjects.

not only required shorter scanning times on average; the length of scanpath and the number of fixations were also considerably reduced. Furthermore, patients showed lower rates of fixation repetitions and larger saccadic amplitudes (see Fig. 2.24 and Table 2.24).

Statistical analysis of eye movement parameters by ANOVA revealed significant ($P < .001$) pre-post differences for scanning time ($F = 256.91$), number of fixations ($F = 149.49$), and fixation repetitions ($F = 309.32$). These differences were also significant ($P < .001$) in each subgroup (scanning time: $F > 112.30$; fixations: $F > 58.58$; fixation repetitions: $F > 124.94$).

Based on these observations the visual search paradigm appears another appropriate means to improve patients' searching and scanning behaviour. This improvement involved the enlargement of saccades as well as the spatiotemporal organisation of oculomotor scanning, resulting in a successful compensation of the visual field defect. Patients' reports on their subjective complaints of problems in everyday life (Table 2.25) is in support of this view. However, a few patients still reported difficulties after practice; these patients also performed worse in the post-treatment tests when compared to the rest of the group. Not surprisingly, these patients suffered from additional injury to the same brain structures as the subgroups mentioned earlier (see p. 59), who also showed inferior performance after treatment. Despite these observations, the visual search paradigm can be evaluated as a highly effective means for the treatment of patients with homonymous field loss to improve their oculomotor compensation strategies. Considering the amount of practice, it appears that patients can benefit more, and certainly earlier when this type of treatment is used. It is, in addition, more flexible with regard to its adaptation to the individual patient, and

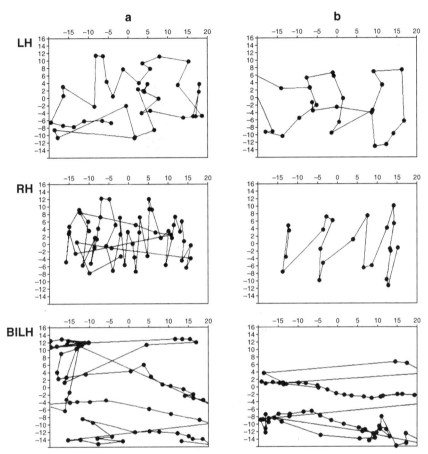

FIG. 2.23 Oculomotor scanning patterns during the scanning of a dot pattern (see Fig. 2.6B) in a patient with left-sided (LH; field sparing = 1°; 9 weeks post-injury), right-sided (RH; field sparing = 2°; 8 weeks), and in a patient with bilateral homonymous hemianopia (BILH; central field sparing = 12°; 11 weeks) before (a) and after (b) practice with visual search. Before practice, the LH patient reported 18 out of 20 dots, the RH patient 17, and the BILH patient 15 dots. After practice, counting was error-free in LH and RH patients; the BILH patient reported 19 dots. Scanning times (in sec): LH: a: 16.9, b: 13.6; RH: a: 22.4, b:19.2; BILH: a: 61.4, b: 43.6. Mean scanning time in a group of 30 age-matched normal control subjects was 9.3 sec (range = 6.2–12.8). Further details as in Fig. 2.18.

has more "motivational impact" because it has more the character of a computer game than of "hard therapeutic" work. Furthermore, we found evidence for transfer of search performance from the smaller to the larger stimulus field. New developments of technology will allow the use of larger projection systems (e.g. beamer systems) in combination with PC software, and thereby improve and enlarge the possibilities of effective training programmes.

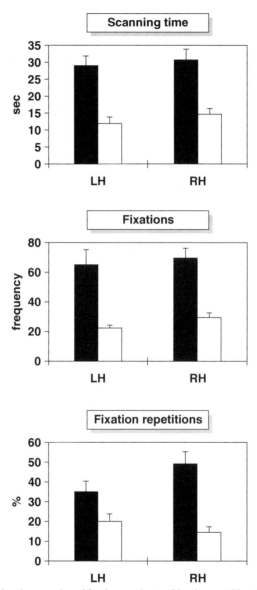

FIG. 2.24 Scanning time, number of fixations, and rate of fixation repetitions in patients with left-sided (LH; $n = 9$) and right-sided (RH; $n = 8$) hemianopia before (dark bars) and after (white bars) practice with visual search. Note decrease in scanning time, number of fixations, and rate of fixation repetition in both patient groups after practice (for corresponding data in nomal subjects, see Table 2.8, p. 39).

TABLE 2.24

Performance in the oculomotor scanning task (counting of 20 dots)
before and after practice with visual search

Group	ST (sec) Before M (1SD)	ST (sec) After M (1SD)	FIX Before M (1SD)	FIX After M (1SD)	FIXr (%) Before M (1SD)	FIXr (%) After M (1SD)
LH (n = 9)	28.8 (5.7)	12.1 (2.7)	62 (16)	25 (8)	46.7 (8.2)	17.4 (11.0)
RH (n = 8)	29.6 (7.9)	14.3 (4.1)	65 (18)	27 (7)	53.9 (12.2)	18.5 (8.6)
N (n = 30)	9.3 (0.8)		23 (4)		12.4 (6.5)	

ST: scanning time; FIX: Fixations; FIXr: repetitions of fixations; LH: patients with left-sided;
RH: with right-sided hemianopia. N: age-matched normal control subjects.

TABLE 2.25

Report of patients with homonymous visual field loss about difficulties in their
everyday life in unfamiliar surroundings before and after practice with visual
search, and at follow up (6–8 weeks post-treatment)

	LH (n = 9) Before	LH (n = 9) After	LH (n = 9) Follow-up	RH (n = 8) Before	RH (n = 8) After	RH (n = 8) Follow-up
Vision "too slow"	9	3	1	8	2	1
Bumping against obstacles	7	1	0	6	2	0
"Getting lost"	4	1	0	3	0	0

LH: patients with left-sided hemianopia; RH: patients with right-sided hemianopia.

Long-term effects

To assess the long-term effects of the treatment procedures described above, we
retested a smaller group of patients (n = 25) 8–12 weeks after the end of training
by recording their eye movements during a scanning task. These patients still
reported some visual difficulties in everyday life at the end of the period of
treatment. In this testing condition a pattern containing 20 dots distributed randomly over the screen was used; the task of the subject was to count the dots (a
parallel version of the task shown in Fig. 2.6B). Figure 2.25 shows oculomotor
scanning patterns in patients with hemianopia and in patients with bilateral field
loss before and after treatment, and at follow-up. As can be seen, all patients
performed similarly at follow-up, indicating that treatment had a positive long-
term effect. Figure 2.26 summarises the follow-up data. On average, scanning
performance was either similar to or even better than performance at the end of
systematic practice with visual scanning on slides (n = 18) or visual search (n = 7).
Thus, patients had used the scanning strategy after systematic practice was finished
and might even have improved through its further use. Patients' subjective

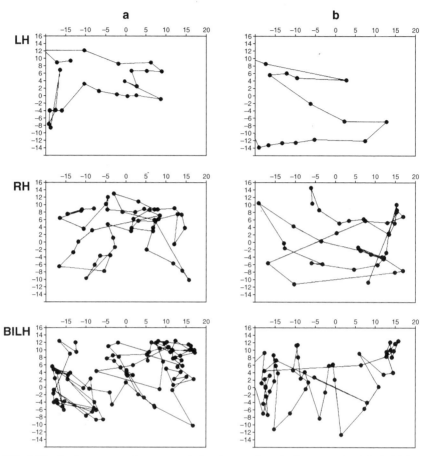

FIG. 2.25   Oculomotor scanning patterns during the scanning of a dot pattern (see Fig. 2.6B) in a patient with left-sided (LH; field sparing = 3°; 8 weeks post-injury), with right-sided (RH; field sparing = 3°; 6 weeks) and with bilateral homonymous hemianopia (BILH; central field sparing = 11°; 8 weeks) after practice (a) with visual search, and at follow-up 8 weeks later (b). Both patients with unilateral hemianopia reported the dots correctly on all testing occasions, while patient BILH reported 17 out of 20 dots after practice and 19 dots at follow-up. Scanning times (in sec): LH: a: 8.9, b: 8.0; RH: a: 18.9, b: 16.9; BILH: a: 55.4, b: 46.7. Further details as in Fig. 2.18.

evaluation of their visual handicap is shown in Table 2.25. The number of patients who complained of difficulties at follow-up was further decreased, but two patients still reported difficulties, for example in crowded places or supermarkets. In conclusion, one can assume that the methods of treatment used were effective in reducing the visual handicap in the majority of patients also in the long-term (see also Kerkhoff, Münssinger, Eberle-Strauss, & Stögerer, 1992a; Kerkhoff et al., 1994).

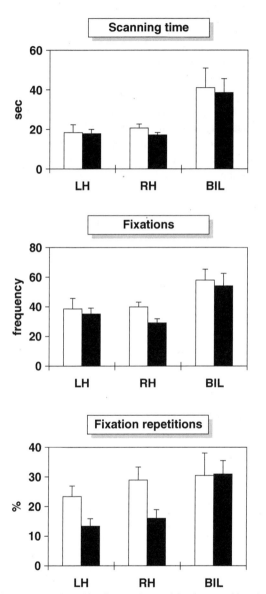

FIG. 2.26 Scanning time, number of fixations, and rate of fixation repetitions in patients with left-sided (LH; $n = 10$), right-sided (RH; $n = 10$), or bilateral (BILH; $n = 5$) hemianopia at the end of practice with visual search (white bars) and at follow-up 8 weeks later (black bars). Note further decrease especially in the rate of fixation repetitions at follow-up in LH and RH patients. For comparison, mean scanning time in a group of 30 age-matched normal control subjects was 9.3sec (range = 6.2–12.8; see also Table 2.8).

TREATMENT OF HEMIANOPIC DYSLEXIA

Reading can be affected after brain injury at various stages of processing (cf. Hillis & Caramazza, 1992). At the visual-sensory level, visual field disorders are the most common cause of reading impairments (Zihl, 1989, 1994). Visual field sparing of less than 5° is typically associated with impaired reading. Since in more than 70% of patients with homonymous field loss field sparing does not exceed 5° (see Table 2.2), this type of reading impairment represents a major source of visual disability in brain-injured people.

It was Wilbrand who in 1907 first described this visual impairment and coined it "macular-hemianopic reading" disorder. He observed that patients with parafoveal (i.e. macular) field loss due to hemianopia, quadranopia, or paracentral scotoma, show rather characteristic reading difficulties that clearly differ from aphasic reading disorders or pure alexia. Patients with left-sided field loss typically have difficulties finding the beginning of a line or a word and very often omit the prefix of polysyllabic words. In contrast, patients with right-sided field loss have great difficulty finding the end of a word and often omit the ending of words. Typically, these patients behave as if "stuck" at that part of the word, they actually look at it and hesitate to move on. Table 2.26 shows examples of

TABLE 2.26
Examples of reading in patients with hemianopic dyslexia: left- (P1)
vs. right-sided (P2) field loss (field sparing = 2°)

Original text
[from: Martin Amis (1994). Career move. In G. Gordon & D. Hughes (Eds.), *The Minerva book of short stories* (p. 14). London: Mandarin Paperbacks.]
The trees were in leaf, and the rumps of the tourist buses were thick and fat in the traffic, and all the farmers wanted fertilizer admixes rather than storehouse insulation when Sixsmith finally made his call. In the interim, Alistair had convinced himself of the following: before returning his aggrieved letter, Sixsmith had steamed it open and then resealed it. During this period also, Alistair had grimly got engaged to Hazel. But the call came.

P1 (LH)
. . . trees were in leaf, and . . . rumps of the tourist uses . . . buses were thick and fat . . . the traffic, and all the . . . farmers wanted fertilizer mixes rather than house insulation when smith finally made his call. In the interim, Alistair had convinced self . . . himself of the following: before turning his grieved . . . aggrieved letter, smith had steamed it open and then sealed . . . sealed it. During this period also, Alistair had grimly got gaged . . . engaged to Hazel. But the call came.

P2 (RH)
The trees were in . . . , and the rumps of . . . tourist buses were thick and fat . . . the traffic, and all . . . farmers want fertile . . . wanted to be fertile . . . admix . . . admixture . . . rather than store . . . insulation when Six . . . finally made his call. In the interim, Ali . . . Alistair had convince . . . to convince . . . himself of the following: before return . . . the return of his aggrieved letter, Six had steamed it open and then resealed it. During this period also, Ali had grimly got engage to Hazel . . . an engagement with Hazel. But the call came.

---

reading of patients with left- and right-sided hemianopia, respectively. Wilbrand (1907) suggested that the parafoveal field loss is the main cause of patients' difficulties with reading, because it prevents their perception of a word as a whole. In free inspection of eye movements in hemianopic patients during reading, Poppelreuter (1917/1990) observed a "disorganised pattern", which no longer consisted of the typical sequence of fixations and small saccadic jumps to the right. These observations were later confirmed by Mackensen (1962), Gassel and Williams (1963a), and Eber et al. (1988) using electro-oculography. Patients with left-sided hemianopia typically show a fragmentation of the return eye movements to the left, while eye movements to the right are smaller and less regular in patients with right-sided hemianopia.

Using infrared-oculography (see p. 23 for a detailed description of the recording technique) we recorded eye movements during reading in patients with parafoveal field loss. The text used consisted of 61 words in 9 lines; unfamiliar and foreign words were avoided. Single lines were vertically separated by 2°. Words were printed in black against a light background (luminance: $0.2cd/m^2$). Letter size was 1°, which is optimal for reading (Legge, Pelli, Rubin, & Schleske, 1985); letter width was 0.5°; spacing between letters was 0.2°. Room illumination was very low (1 lux). Subjects were asked to read the text silently, with no further instructions on how to proceed, and had to provide a report on the content of the text afterwards. Recording was started at the onset of text presentation and was ended after the subject indicated completion of reading. A fixation was defined by a spatial window of 1.5° and a duration of 100msec. Eye movement data were quantitatively analysed with respect to total reading time, number and amplitude of saccades, number and duration of fixations, and repetition rates of fixations.

Figures 2.27 and 2.28 show examples of reading eye movements in normal subjects and in patients with uni- and bilateral parafoveal field disorders. Normal subjects showed the typical staircase pattern in the direction of reading (i.e. from left to right). The patient with left-sided hemianopia mainly had difficulties shifting fixation accurately from the end of a line to the beginning of the next line. In contrast, the patient with right-sided hemianopia found it extremely difficult to guide his eyes from the beginning of a line to its end. His eye shifts were irregular, with a high number of regressive saccades and many fixation repetitions. Similar alterations of reading eye movements were found in patients with unilateral left- and right-sided paracentral scotoma and with hemiamblyopia involving the parafoveal region. Patients with bilateral parafoveal visual field loss or bilateral hemiamblyopia showed, as one would expect, a combination of the alterations found in cases with left- and right-sided field loss, i.e. they had difficulties finding the beginning of a line accurately and guiding their eyes rightward from the beginning to the end of the line.

That the alterations in the reading eye movement patterns reflect patients' reading impairment is shown in Table 2.27. Reading performance, defined as

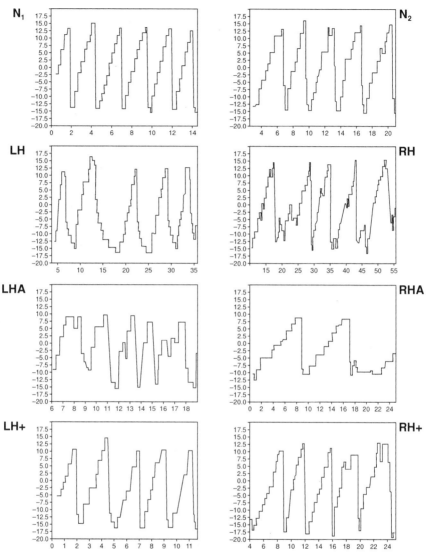

FIG. 2.27 Reading eye movements in two normal control subjects (N1: "good" reader, N2: "poor" reader), patients with left-sided (LH; field sparing = 1°; 7 weeks post-injury) and right-sided hemianopia (RH; field sparing = 2°; 6 weeks), and in patients with left-sided hemiamblyopia (LHA; field sparing = 2°; 6 weeks), and with right-sided hemiamblyopia (RHA; field sparing = 3°; 5 weeks). LH+, RH+: reading eye movements in patients with left- and right-sided hemianopia (field sparing = 2°; 6 and 7 weeks post-injury) with moderate hemianopic dyslexia. x-axis: time period of recording (in sec), y-axis: horizontal extension of line (in degrees). 0 = centre, negative values left, positive values right. Subjects were asked to read silently five lines of text (RHA: 3 lines). Note difficulties of fixation shifting to the left in LH and LHA patients, and the increased number of regressive fixations in RH and RHA patients. Reading performance (words per minute): N1: 151, N2: 95; LH: 57; RH: 39; LHA: 87, RHA: 72; LH+: 145, RH+: 86. For comparison, mean reading performance in a group of 25 normal subjects was 174 wpm (range = 139–237).

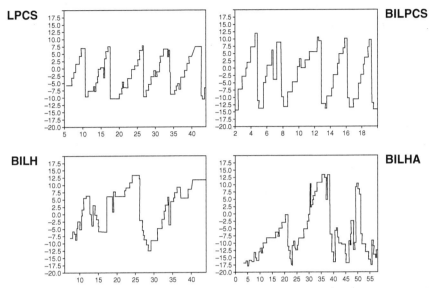

LPCS   **BILPCS**

BILH   **BILHA**

FIG. 2.28   Reading eye movements in patients with left-sided paracentral scotoma (LPCS; field sparing = 2°; 5 weeks post-injury), bilateral paracentral scotoma (BILPCS; central field sparing = 5°; 8 weeks), bilateral hemianopia (BILH; sparing = 7°; 8 weeks), and with bilateral hemiamblyopia (BILHA; sparing = 6°; 7 weeks). Note difficulties in guiding fixation systematically in all patients, and loss of orientation within lines in cases with bilateral field loss (BILH, BILHA; only two text lines). Reading performance (words per minute): LPCS: 98, BILPCS: 44; BILH: 19, BILHA: 12. For further details, see Fig. 2.27.

correctly read words per minute (wpm; the text consisted of 180 words in 20 lines; Univers, 12pt, 1.5 line spacing), is markedly reduced in patients as compared to age-matched normal subjects. In addition, patients with right-sided parafoveal field loss showed a considerably lower reading rate compared to patients with left-sided parafoveal field loss. This difference can be explained by the left-to-right orthography (Zihl, 1995a).

Thus, earlier and recent observations strongly suggest that parafoveal field loss affects reading at the sensory level; it prevents the patient from perceiving a word as a whole and impairs the visual guidance of eye movements. It is well known that the parafoveal field region plays a crucial role in both text recognition and guidance of eye movements in reading (e.g. Rayner & Pollatsek, 1987; Rayner, McConkie, & Ehrlich, 1978). The fovea possesses the highest acuity and the resolving power required for discrimination and identification of letters and numbers. Although visual acuity decreases sharply with increasing eccentricity (Anstis, 1974), the parafoveal region allows gross feature information processing, as for example the length of words (Ikeda & Saida, 1978; Inhoff, 1987). Thus, both the foveal and the parafoveal field regions act as a common "perceptual window" and provide the basis for the so-called reading span, which is defined as the field of useful vision in reading during an eye fixation (McConkie

TABLE 2.27

Reading performance in 152 patients with uni- and 13 patients with
bilateral visual field disorders and visual field sparing < 5°

Group	n	Words read correctly per minute M (range)	No. of patients complaining of reading difficulties n (%)
Unilateral visual field disorders			
LH	64	78 (33–141)	49 (76.6)
RH	51	56 (14–94)	46 (90.2)
LQ	6	109 (79–148)	3
RQ	6	76 (50–96)	5
LPCS	6	90 (43–140)	3
RPCS	5	68 (34–85)	4
LHA	5	81 (43–103)	3
RHA	9	56 (27–97)	7
Bilateral field disorders			
BILH	3	42 (27–59)	3
BILHA	3	54 (44–62)	3
BILPCS	7	51 (31–98)	6
N	25	174 (139–237)	

LH, RH: patients with left- or right hemianopia; LQ, RQ: patients with left- or right-sided quadranopia; LPCS, RPCS: patients with left- or right-sided paracentral scotoma; LHA, RHA: patients with left- or right-sided hemianopia; BILH, BILHA: patients with bilateral hemianopia or hemiamblyopia; BILPCS: patients with bilateral paracentral scotomata. N: age-matched normal subjects.

& Rayner, 1975, 1976). The eye movement data we obtained from patients with parafoveal field loss underline the importance of this visual field region for the processing of words as a whole and for the visual guidance of eye movements during reading. Table 2.28 summarises the results of the quantitative analysis of the oculomotor reading pattern in 79 patients with unilateral or bilateral field defects. When compared to normal subjects, patients with left- and right-sided hemianopia show not only longer reading times, but also more and longer fixations, a higher percentage of refixations, and smaller saccadic amplitudes. Not unexpectedly, patients with right-sided field loss showed a more severe impairment than patients with left-sided hemianopia. The degree of reduction in reading performance appears to depend mainly on the extent of visual field sparing, as Table 2.29 shows. Patients with only 1–2° of sparing showed the poorest performance with right-sided hemianopic patients performing worst. When 4° of the parafoveal field are spared, patients with left-sided hemianopia showed, on average, nearly normal reading performance. Patients with right-sided hemianopia, however, required at least 6° of sparing for "normal" reading. The subjective complaints of patients are in agreement with this observation. Patients with at least 4–5° of field sparing, who showed normal or nearly normal reading

TABLE 2.28
Eye movement parameters during reading of a text of 48 words in 69 patients
with unilateral and in 10 patients with bilateral parafoveal visual field loss

Group	n	FIX M (1SD)	FIXr (%) M (1SD)	FD (sec) M (1SD)	A (°) M (1SD)
Unilateral field disorders					
LH	29	76 (15)	36.5 (14.2)	0.31 (0.08)	4.0 (1.1)
RH	27	87 (23)	44.4 (17.8)	0.41 (0.17)	3.2 (1.4)
LQ	2	65	28.6	0.26	4.1
RQ	1	81	44.7	0.36	3.4
LPCS	4	72	22.5	0.27	4.0
RPCS	1	87	26.1	0.28	3.7
LHA	1	69	40.4	0.28	4.1
RHA	4	94	44.8	0.37	3.8
Bilateral field disorders					
BILH	3	136	64.6	0.49	2.9
BILHA	3	122	47.8	0.35	3.1
BILPCS	4	116	53.1	0.47	3.4
N	25	56 (11)	15.2 (9.6)	0.25 (0.02)	4.3 (0.7)

FIX: number of fixations, FIXr: repetition of fixations, FD: fixation durations, A: saccadic
amplitudes in the direction of reading (left to right). Other abbreviations as in Table 2.27.

TABLE 2.29
Reading performance in 144 patients with unilateral hemianopia and
different degrees of visual field sparing (VFSP)

Group	VFSP	n	Words read correctly per minute M (range)	No. of patients complaining of reading difficulty n (%)
LH	< 3°	36	53 (33–79)	29 (80.6)
	3–5°	28	74 (51–108)	12 (42.9)
	> 5°	13	124 (96–162)	2 (15.4)
RH	< 3°	31	43 (14–53)	29 (93.6)
	3–5°	20	58 (47–84)	14 (70.0)
	> 5°	16	98 (77–116)	6 (37.5)
N		25	174 (139–237)	

LH, RH: patients with left- or right hemianopia. N: normal control subjects.

performance also reported, as a rule, only mild difficulties with reading.
However, there is a small group of patients who showed and reported "normal"
reading performance in spite of only 1–2° of field sparing. These patients also
showed quite normal oculomotor reading patterns (Fig. 2.27). Since time since
brain injury, age, and "premorbid" reading performance (calculated on the basis

of school education levels) did not differ considerably between this subgroup and the other patients, another factor must be responsible for this difference. In searching for this factor we found that patients with injury to the optic radiation or the striate cortex without additional involvement of the white matter, occipitoparietal structures, or the posterior thalamus showed very effective spontaneous compensation, while patients suffering from additional injury to these structures did not (Zihl, 1995a). Gassel and Williams (1963a) reported that about 30% of their 35 hemianopic patients no longer exhibited oculomotor abnormalities during reading when followed over a period of years, i.e. this subgroup of patients had eventually successfully adapted to their field loss. In our group, time since brain injury was much shorter (6 weeks on average; range = 3–12 weeks) and only 8 out of 50 patients (16%) showed effective spontaneous compensation. Of course, one is inclined to assume that a longer follow-up would have increased the number of patients with successful (spontaneous) oculomotor compensation also in our group. In conclusion, these observations suggest that the visual field sparing does not appear to be the only factor causing persistent hemianopic dyslexia, but also the extent of brain injury (Zihl, 1995a), a factor that has also been found to play a crucial role in visual scanning (see p. 59).

Proceeding from these observations and based on the considerations concerning the roles of the parafoveal visual field, visual attention, and spatial guidance of eye movements in reading, we developed methods of treatment that were supposed to give patients with parafoveal field loss specific practice with reading. It is important to recall here which kind of difficulties patients with left- or right-sided parafoveal field loss exhibit. Both groups begin too early with the semantic processing (i.e. extraction of the meaning) of the text material they have seen, in spite of missing text information to the left or right of the fixation point. Therefore, the main focus of the treatment procedure was the shift of fixation (and, of course, attention) either to the beginning of each word, including the one at the beginning of a new line, or to the end of each word. In principle, the missing parafoveal field was expected to be substituted by adapting the oculomotor pattern to the altered condition of visual processing of text material. As a result, visual text information processing should possibly be regained at this "lower" level of reading.

Practice using an electronic reading aid

In a first series of investigations (Zihl, 1988, 1990; Zihl, Krischer, & Meissen, 1984) we used a computer-based electronic aid to improve patients' reading performance. This reading aid consisted of a monitor (a 70 × 50cm television screen) and a microcomputer that allowed the generation and presentation of text information. To reduce the difficulty of reading, especially when several lines of text are presented (as, for example, in a book or a newspaper), only one line of text was shown at a time. Since the direction of reading in our subjects was left to right, the text moved smoothly from right to left to make text apprehension easier. We hypothesised that the regaining of appropriate guidance of reading eye movements could be improved and accelerated by the movement of the text towards the actual location of the fovea from the right to the left edge of the screen. The speed of the moving text, the height and spacing of characters, and foreground and background colours could be varied. Usually yellow text was presented against a blue or black background. Reading texts varied from single words with different length to short stories.

A group of 120 patients with homonymous field disorders affecting the parafoveal region participated in this study. The majority of patients (74%) showed homonymous hemianopia; field sparing ranged from 1° to 5°, with a mean of 2.6°. All patients suffered from vascular lesions in the postchiasmatic visual system, mainly due to infarctions in the territory of the posterior cerebral arteries. Time since brain injury was on average 6.3 weeks (range = 3–18 weeks). Reading performance before and after practice was assessed using parallel versions of a text consisting of 180 words (Univers, 12pt) in 20 lines (1.5 line spacing). Before treatment, all patients exhibited impaired reading, i.e. reading performance was lower than the mean of a group of normal control subjects plus 3 standard deviations (2.2min for 180 words; 1 uncorrected reading error at maximum). After treatment, the majority of patients (78%) showed "normal" reading, i.e. reading speed and number of reading errors were within the ranges of normal control subjects. Patients with right-sided field loss required considerably more sessions (mean = 34; range = 17–46) of practice than patients with left-sided field loss (mean = 24; range = 12–29). Furthermore, patients with field sparing of less than 3° on average required more practice than patients with more than 3° of sparing, irrespective of the side of field loss. It should be added that in 42 out of the 120 patients (35%) we found an enlargement of the visual field by 2–3° (mean = 2.4°) after practice. This increase was only found along the horizontal meridian and is in agreement with findings reported by Kerkhoff et al. (1992a).

As already mentioned, after treatment, the majority of patients (78%) showed a significant improvement of their reading performance. However, the percentage of patients reporting an improvement in reading was lower (63%). One factor influencing the subjective evaluation of the improvement in reading is, of course, the "premorbid" level of reading performance. Patients who reported having been highly skilled readers (academics, especially teachers) reported less improvement despite the same amount of treatment and the same degree of improvement. They still complained of partly severe reading impairment and felt equally handicapped after treatment, having achieved no real amelioration. In contrast, patients with lower educational level reported marked improvement in their reading ability and were highly satisfied with the outcome of treatment. They also evaluated their improved reading clearly as an improvement in their life quality. Extreme examples are the cases of a 46-year-old bricklayer and a 48-year-old teacher. The bricklayer told us that after practice, which increased his reading performance from 36wpm to 96wpm, he now finds reading quite exciting and pleasant. He had begun, therefore, not only to read newspapers regularly, but had also started, probably for the first time in his life, to read books. In contrast, the teacher, although he could read fluently again (his reading performance improved from 64 wpm before to 113 wpm after practice), insisted that his reading performance had not been improved after practice, "I cannot read at the same speed as in earlier times and any reading below my (earlier) personal level is not real reading in my view". Quite understandably, this patient did not evaluate the improvement in reading as a real improvement in his life quality. These examples show that the level of "premorbid" reading performance plays a crucial role in the subjective judgement of reading performance after treatment and of its impact on life quality.

As in the case of oculomotor scanning and searching (see p. 48 and p. 61) we found again two subgroups of patients with respect to the effectiveness of treatment. As mentioned above, the majority of cases (78%) benefited from the treatment to such an extent that their reading performance after practice was within the normal range. A smaller group of cases (22%), in contrast, required more training sessions and nevertheless exhibited less improvement at the end of the treatment period. These patients, in addition to the injury to the postchiasmatic visual pathway, showed extensive injury to the occipital white matter and to occipitoparietal regions and/or to the posterior thalamus. It appears, therefore, that injury to these posterior brain structures not only prevents effective spontaneous adaptation to the field defect, but also can impair the acquisition of compensatory reading strategies by systematic practice (Zihl, 1995a).

Follow-up measurements 6–8 weeks after the end of treatment revealed a further improvement in reading speed. However, patients with extensive posterior brain injury still performed worse even 8 weeks after treatment, although they also reported to have read daily, as instructed, for at least 30 minutes.

Summarising these observations it can be concluded that hemianopic dyslexia can be successfully treated. The improvement took place during the period of treatment, and was accompanied by the adaptation of the oculomotor reading pattern to the parafoveal field loss. Thus, the improved reading can be explained by the substitution of the lost parafoveal field region by saccadic eye movements (Zihl, 1995a). The observation that reading performance did not deteriorate after the end of systematic practice indicates that the effect of training was stable and persistent. The continued regular reading at home had led to a further improvement, which was, however, not as pronounced as was the improvement observed after systematic and specific practice in the training period. Similar observations have been reported by Kerkhoff et al. (1992a) in a group of 56 patients with parafoveal field loss. In conclusion, there is convincing evidence that hemianopic dyslexia can be treated successfully.

PC-based tachistoscopic presentation of text material

Although the method of treatment described in the last section has proved to be useful in the rehabilitation of patients with reading impairment due to parafoveal visual field loss, it has two disadvantages. First, the electronic reading aid is mainly hardware-based and therefore has limited flexibility. Second, the amount of training was quite high, especially in patients with right-sided field loss. We therefore searched for an alternative method which combines higher flexibility with lower costs. These prerequisites could be realised by means of a software program which allows time-limited (tachistoscopic) presentation of text material in a highly flexible manner. Files with text units can be produced easily by the therapist according to the individual severity of the hemianopic dyslexia. Presentation time can be varied such that the patient can get immediate feedback on whether he or she has seen the whole word or not. This feedback was expected to force the patient to move the fixation more efficiently, i.e. as quickly as possible to either the beginning or the end of a word, depending on the side of the field loss. The use of a 17-inch high-resolution monitor enables sufficiently high quality of text presentation of words in the centre, to the left and to the right of the centre of the screen (Fig. 2.29). In addition, the size and colour of the words can be varied as well as the colour of the background. We usually chose yellow for the text and a dark blue for the background. Room illumination was low (< 5 lux) to help prevent blinding effects on the monitor.

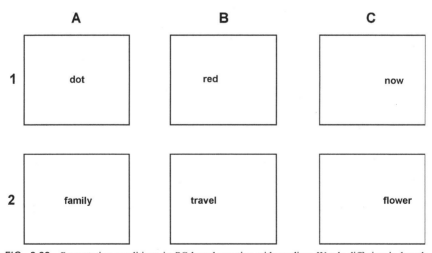

FIG. 2.29 Presentation conditions in PC-based practice with reading. Words differing in length (1, 2) were presented either in the centre (A), or left (B) or right (C) of centre. B and C were used after patients with left- or right-sided parafoveal field loss were able to read correctly in condition A.

The procedure of the treatment was typically as follows: In the beginning, shorter (3–4 letters) and longer (4–7 letters) words were used and were presented for 1000, 750, and later 500msec. At the beginning of the treatment, words were always presented in the centre of the monitor. To enhance fixation shifts, words were later either presented to the left (in cases with left-sided field defects) or right of centre (in cases with right-sided field defects). In the last stage of practice, words were presented in random order in the centre, or to the left or right of it. Presentation time was reduced when a patient was able to read words of a given length correctly. In the second phase, short (2–3 words) sentences (e.g. "a red apple", "the playing child") were used, with presentation time being reduced from 1500 to 750 or even to 500msec. In the third phase, longer phrases (4–6 words) were used; presentation time was 2000, 1500, 1000, and eventually 750msec.

As with the previous method of treatment, patients with left-sided field loss were instructed to search as quickly as possible for the beginning of a word, while patients with right-sided field loss should search as quickly as possible for the ending of a word. Patients were informed that words would disappear before they had read them if they were too slow in shifting their eyes to the beginning or end of the words, respectively.

A group of 32 patients suffering from uni- or bilateral paracentral field defects (see Table 2.30) was trained according to this method. Pre- and post-treatment reading performance was assessed using parallel versions of a text consisting of 180 words (Univers, 12 pt) in 20 lines. Patients showed neither visual neglect nor pure or aphasic dyslexia. Table 2.31 shows reading performance before and after treatment, and the number of training sessions. While reading speed was increased, the number of errors was decreased after training in both groups. Statistical analysis (ANOVA) of data revealed a significant treatment effect for reading performance (words per minute; $F = 106.01$; $P < .001$). The significant

TABLE 2.30
Treatment with tachistoscopic word presentation: Demographical data
of 32 patients with homonymous visual field loss

Group	n	Gender (M/F)	Age (years) M (range)	T (weeks) M (range)	VFSP (°) M (range)
LH	12	1/11	56 (41–79)	18 (9–38)	2.1 (1–3)
RH	7	3/4	48 (21–66)	14 (9–22)	2.3 (1–4)
LQ	3	0/3	45 (28–72)	12 (9–14)	2.3 (1–3)
LPCS	1	0/1	41	11	2.0
RHA	3	0/3	28 (18–46)	19 (15–26)	3.0 (2–4)
BILH	2	0/2	62 (60,64)	13 (10,16)	6* (5,7)
BILHA	2	1/1	51 (43,58)	12 (11,13)	7* (6,8)
BILPCS	2	0/2	57 (54,60)	17 (16,18)	5* (4,6)

Abbreviations as in Table 2.28. T: time since brain injury, VFSP: visual field sparing
*diameter of spared central visual field.

TABLE 2.31

Results of reading performance before and after practice using tachistoscopic presentation in 26 patients with unilateral and in 6 patients with bilateral parafoveal field loss (cf. Table 2.30)

Group	Words per minute		Uncorrected errors		Sessions	Trials
	Before	After	Before	After		
LH (n = 12)						
M (range)	82 (38–128)	114 (75–151)	2.8 (2–5)	0.3 (0–1)	7 (4–11)	1650 (920–2760)
RH (n = 7)						
M (range)	67 (39–90)	113 (75–153)	4.4 (3–7)	0.6 (0–2)	9 (7–14)	2360 (1380–3040)
LQ1	81	119	5	0	11	2080
LQ2	116	150	0	0	6	1560
LQ3	78	109	6	2	12	2380
LPCS	104	164	2	0	5	1050
RHA1	86	138	7	2	8	2110
RHA2	54	88	5	0	8	1750
RHA3	53	84	4	1	7	1680
BILH1	21	43	9	3	16	3440
BILH2	27	64	11	2	14	3280
BILHA1	64	99	7	1	12	2820
BILHA2	30	51	6	2	11	2560
BILPCS1	81	126	3	0	9	2250
BILPCS2	23	38	5	1	10	2660
N	174 (139–237)					

Between 190 and 260 trials per session were carried out. Abbreviations as in Table 2.28. For the LH- and RH-patients means and ranges are shown; for the other patient groups the individual values are given. N: mean reading performance of 25 normal control subjects for comparison.

increase in reading performance was found in patients with left- and patients with right-sided hemianopia ($F > 35.08$; $P < .001$).

Reading performance was somewhat lower in patients with right-sided field defects (mean = 109 wpm; range = 75–153) than in patients with left-sided field defects (mean = 119 wpm; range = 75–164), although the difference did not reach statistical significance. As with the former training technique, patients with right-sided field defects required more practice sessions (mean = 10, range = 7–14) than patients with left-sided defects (mean = 8; range = 4–12). However, a smaller number of sessions was required to improve patients' reading ability compared with the treatment using the electronic reading aid (number of sessions in patients with left-sided field defects mean = 24, range = 12–29; in patients with right-sided field defects mean = 34, range = 17–46). Thus, the method using tachistoscopic presentation of text material appears to have accelerated the acquisition of a successful oculomotor compensation strategy in both groups.

The improvement in reading performance was again accompanied by corresponding changes in the oculomotor reading pattern (Fig. 2.30) and also in the various quantitative oculomotor parameters (see Table 2.32). For the statistical analysis of oculomotor parameters by ANOVA both groups of patients were combined. The analysis revealed significant ($P < .001$) pre-post differences for the number of fixations ($F = 31.76$), the number of fixation repetitions ($F = 44.69$), fixation duration ($F = 24.75$), and the size of saccadic shifts to the right ($F = 23.57$). Thus, after practice, the number of fixations was significantly reduced, the duration of fixations significantly shorter, and the amplitudes of saccades to the right significantly larger.

Using the same method of reading practice, we also treated six patients with bilateral parafoveal field loss. Because of their "bilateral" problem in reading, these patients had to search both for the beginning and for the end of each word before reading it. The outcome of treatment in this group of patients is shown in Table 2.31. Again, we found a considerable improvement in reading, both with respect to the speed of reading and the number of reading errors. Recording of eye movements revealed that the oculomotor reading pattern showed the expected changes (Fig. 2.31). After treatment, patients showed larger saccades and less fixations, and used shorter fixation durations (Table 2.32). Patients with bilateral parafoveal field loss required more practice (12 sessions on average) than patients with unilateral field loss (8 sessions on average). Nevertheless, they also benefited from this type of training.

Reading impairment in patients with uni- or bilateral homonymous hemiamblyopia was treated in a similar way as in patients with uni- or bilateral hemianopia. Table 2.31 shows the outcome of treatment in three patients with right-sided and in two cases with bilateral hemiamblyopia. After seven to eight sessions these patients showed a considerable improvement in reading, which was also reflected by their oculomotor reading patterns (Figs. 2.30 and 2.31, and Table 2.32). The degree of improvement in reading and the number of training

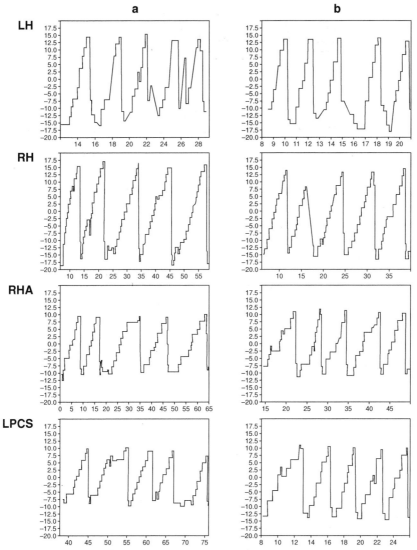

FIG. 2.30 Reading eye movements in patients with unilateral paracentral field loss before (a) and after (b) practice. LH: patient with left-sided hemianopia (field sparing = 2°; beginning of practice: 7 weeks post-injury); RH: patient with right-sided hemianopia (sparing = 1°; 6 weeks); LHA: patient with left-sided hemiamblyopia (sparing = 2°; 7 weeks); RHA: patient with right-sided hemiamblyopia (sparing = 3°; 7 weeks); LPCS: patient right-sided paracentral scotoma (sparing = 2°; 6 weeks). Note improvement in the pattern of reading eye movements after practice in all patients. Reading performance (words per minute): LH: a: 102, b: 138; RH: a: 35, b: 53; LHA: a: 97, b: 120; RHA: a: 27, b: 51; RPCS: a: 47, b: 99. For comparison, mean reading performance in a group of 25 normal subjects was 174 wpm (range: 139–237). For further details, see Fig. 2.27.

TABLE 2.32

Reading eye movement parameters (48 words) before and after practice with reading in 16 patients with unilateral and in 3 patients with bilateral parafoveal visual field loss (cf. Table 2.30)

Group	FIX	FIXr (%)	FD (sec)	A (°)
LH (n = 6)				
M (range)				
before	80 (52–112)	25.1 (12.7–37.8)	0.29 (0.24–0.32)	3.8 (3.2–4.4)
after	64 (33–95)	17.9 (3.7–35.6)	0.25 (0.24–0.27)	4.6 (4.3–5.0)
RH (n = 5)				
M (range)				
before	98 (73–125)	42.1 (22.4–75.6)	0.43 (0.28–0.50)	2.9 (2.7–3.3)
after	77 (57–109)	33.7 (11.8–65.4)	0.33 (0.26–0.42)	3.2 (2.7–3.6)
LQ (n = 3)				
M (range)				
before	67 (48–91)	17.2 (9.8–24.4)	0.27 (0.24–0.29)	4.2 (3.9–4.5)
after	56 (54–72)	14.6 (7.8–20.0)	0.25 (0.24–0.26)	4.7 (4.4–5.1)
PCSL				
before	78	23.1	0.26	3.5
after	57	19.3	0.24	4.6
HA				
before	170	45.5	0.45	2.6
after	88	25.9	0.38	2.8
BILH				
before	165	63.0	0.36	2.8
after	108	39.8	0.28	4.3
BILHA				
before	143	51.7	0.34	3.4
after	83	38.6	0.26	4.1
BILPCS				
before	102	36.3	0.35	3.7
after	62	14.5	0.28	4.7
N (n = 25)				
M (range)	54 (23–42)	15.8 (1.8–11.6)	0.24 (0.20–0.28)	4.4 (3.6–5.2)

FIX: number of fixations, FIXr: repetition of fixations, FD: fixation durations, A: saccadic amplitudes in the direction of reading (left to right). Abbreviations as in Table 2.28. For the LH, RH, and LQ patients means and ranges are shown; for the other patients the individual values are given. N: age-matched normal subjects, for comparison.

sessions were indeed comparable to the corresponding numbers in patients with right-sided or bilateral hemianopia. This again indicates that the loss of form vision in the parafoveal field region can affect reading in a similar way as the total loss of vision in this part of the visual field, and that the same type of treatment can reduce this visual impairment.

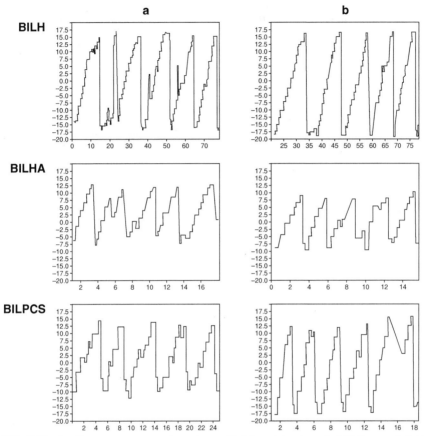

FIG. 2.31 Reading eye movements in patients with bilateral hemianopia (BILH; central field sparing = 4°; 9 weeks post-injury), with bilateral hemiamblyopia (BILHA; sparing = 6°; 8 weeks), and with bilateral paracentral scotoma (BILPCS; central field sparing = 4°) before (a) and after (b) practice. Reading performance (words per minute): BILH: a: 21, b: 31; BILHA: a: 106; b: 123; BILPCS: a: 75, b: 103. Further details as in Fig. 2.27.

We asked patients before and after treatment to evaluate their difficulties with reading. Table 2.33 shows the results. As expected, patients with right-sided field loss reported more frequent and more severe difficulties before treatment. After treatment, the majority of patients reported a distinct improvement in their ability to read. A small group that mainly corresponded to the group of patients with additional injury to the posterior brain still reported mild or moderate difficulties.

All patients were encouraged to continue reading regularly at home. Follow-up testing 8 weeks after the end of training revealed further improvement in reading performance, and reading eye movements reflected this further improvement (Fig. 2.32). Thus, patients can retain their level of reading performance when they further use their regained reading capacity.

TABLE 2.33

Reports of 32 patients with homonymous visual field loss
(cf. Table 2.30) about difficulties with reading before and after
practice, and at follow up (6–8 weeks post-treatment)

Group	Before practice No. of patients	After practice No. of patients	Follow-up No. of patients
UNIL (n = 16)	16	2	1
UNIR (n = 10)	10	4	1
BIL (n = 6)	6	3	2

UNIL, UNIR: patients with left- and with right-sided unilateral field defects (hemianopia, quadranopia, paracentral scotoma, hemiamblyopia); BIL: patients with bilateral parafoveal field defects.

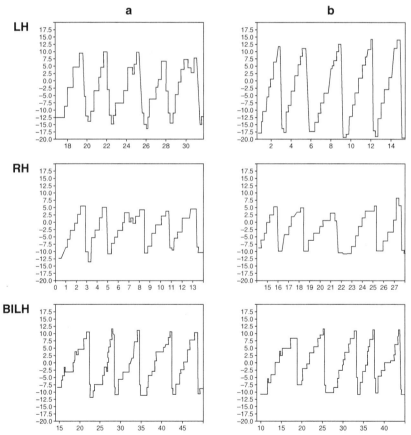

FIG. 2.32   Reading eye movements in patients with left-sided (LH; sparing = 3°), right-sided (RH; sparing = 3°), and bilateral hemianopia (BILH; sparing of central field = 6°) at the end of practice (a) and 8 weeks later at follow-up testing (b). Reading performance (words per minute): LH: a: 53, b: 75; RH: a: 61, b: 66; BILH: a: 33, b: 37. Further details as in Fig. 2.27.

In conclusion, the method of tachistoscopic word and text presentation appears even more effective for the treatment of patients with hemianopic dyslexia than the method reported in the foregoing section, because patients required less practice to regain reading. This especially holds true for patients with right-sided parafoveal field loss, who on average showed a similar reading performance after treatment as patients with left-sided field loss. The high flexibility of the program allows the composition of highly individual training programmes, it can easily be used by the therapist and is far less expensive than the first method. In short, this method fulfils even more the essential requirements of a useful and widely acceptable treatment procedure in the rehabilitation of patients with hemianopic dyslexia.

It should be emphasised here that the recording of eye movements was a very helpful tool to demonstrate and specify precisely the abnormalities of reading patterns associated with the parafoveal field loss (see also Ciuffreda, Kenyon, & Stark, 1985). Furthermore, the analysis of reading eye movements before and after practice enabled us to measure and understand the adaptive processes underlying the improvement in reading, and thus, also allowed a more objective assessment of practice effects.

OPTICAL AIDS AND HEAD SHIFTS

Optical aids (mirror systems or prism systems) that substitute the lost visual field have been described by several authors. Reports about the efficacy and usefulness of such aids, however, are controversial. While some authors (Igersheimer, 1919; Rossi, Kheyfets, & Reding, 1990; Weiss, 1969, 1972) found these aids to be somewhat useful, others did not (Teuber et al., 1960). For the moment, it appears difficult to find convincing arguments in favour or disfavour of these aids. Optical aids are expensive; their fitting is very time-consuming and requires special efforts by both the patient and the therapist. It is only after intensive practice that a patient might experience some benefit. Furthermore, the mirror reversal of the visual image can cause serious difficulties when the patient is shifting the gaze or is walking. Gaze shifts may disorganise the patient's visual perception to the point that nausea is induced. The patient has to learn to use only a special section of the prism while walking. To change fixation, the patient must stop walking, make the fixation change, and then continue walking (Weiss, 1972). Rossi et al. (1990) described in more detail the outcome of using diopter plastic homonymous Fresnel prisms in patients with hemianopia. The prism-treated group performed significantly better on visuospatial tests, but no functional benefit in daily life could be demonstrated. In conclusion, optical aids represent an interesting possibility for the remediation of hemianopic patients' visual handicap at least in some conditions, but further studies are required to test their usefulness and to gain criteria indicating who will benefit from them.

Patients with hemianopia or other homonymous field defects are often told to shift their head towards the affected side and to keep it there in order to overcome the field loss. If one considers the normal physiological sequence of head and eye movements, then this instruction appears obsolete. Head movements usually follow eye movements and head displacements depend on the amplitude and temporal course of the saccadic movements (Uemura et al., 1980). Considering eye–head co-ordination in oculomotor scanning and in fixating objects, reversing this order to compensate for hemianopia certainly does not contribute to effective gaze shifts (Zangemeister et al., 1982) and may even have a detrimental effect on visual exploration and reading (Kerkhoff et al., 1992a,b).

CHAPTER THREE

Disorders in visual acuity, spatial contrast sensitivity, and visual adaptation

Visual acuity is usually not particularly impaired after unilateral postchiasmatic brain injury except in cases where the optic tract is involved. In contrast, spatial contrast sensitivity and visual adaptation can be impaired after unilateral postchiasmatic injury and can affect visual capacities that demand high spatial resolution, as in reading for example. In patients with impaired spatial contrast vision, visual acuity may be unaffected if tested using high-contrast single optotypes. Nevertheless, these patients are visually disabled as described in more detail later.

VISUAL ACUITY

In patients with unilateral injury to the optic tract, visual acuity may be reduced either in the eye ipsilateral to the site of brain injury or in both eyes (Savino, Paris, Schatz, & Corbett, 1978). However, as Frisén (1980) has argued, a relative acuity of 90%, for example, evaluated as being within the normal range, may in fact already represent a reduction, because the (usually not exactly known) relative acuity of a patient prior to brain injury might have been 100% or even higher. Thus, visual acuity levels below 100%, which are not due to peripheral factors and cannot be improved by optical correction, may be caused by unilateral postchiasmatic brain injury. Whether or not this reduction represents a visual handicap depends on whether further visual dysfunctions (e.g. contrast vision) are present or not. Patients with bilateral postchiasmatic brain injury may show normal visual acuity, but they can also exhibit a severe reduction in acuity up to crude form vision (Pöppel et al., 1978; Symonds & MacKenzie, 1957).

91

SPATIAL CONTRAST SENSITIVITY

Patients with acquired posterior brain injury sometimes complain of "blurred" or "foggy" vision in the presence of normal visual acuity, accommodation, and convergence (for a review on "blurred vision" and its various causes, see Walsh, 1985). The measurement of spatial contrast sensitivity has been found to be useful to understand better visual impairment in tasks involving a high resolution capacity of the visual system, as for example in reading or fine form discrimination. As mentioned above, impaired spatial resolution is not necessarily always associated with a reduction in visual acuity. By measuring visual acuity alone one would therefore be unable to uncover the underlying deficit (Acheson & Sanders, 1995; Arden, 1978; Hess, 1984).

Spatial contrast sensitivity is usually assessed by measuring monocular or binocular contrast detection thresholds for black–white grating stimuli ranging from 0.5 to 50 cycles/degree (c/deg). The grating stimuli are presented on a raster display, with spatial frequency (i.e. width and spatial separation of black–white bars) and contrast between bars being varied independently. The subject's task is to detect the particular grating while the contrast is stepwise increased or decreased (Bodis-Wollner & Diamond, 1976; Bulens, Meerwaldt, van der Wildt, & Kemink, 1989; Hess, Zihl, Pointer, & Schmid, 1990).

We used a Joyce Electronics (Cambridge, UK) raster display (white P4 phosphor) for the presentation of vertical sinusoidal gratings. Gratings were generated and presented and responses collected and analysed using a microcomputer. The mean screen luminance was $100cd/m^2$ and the frame rate was 100Hz. The contrast linearity of the display screen allowed up to 98% contrast. At a viewing distance of 6m the screen subtended 6° horizontally and 4° vertically. Monocular and binocular contrast thresholds were measured under mesopic viewing conditions using a two-alternative, forced-choice technique. The subject had to detect the presence of the vertical grating pattern in one half of the screen and to indicate its presence by either pressing the left or right response key in correspondence with the side of the appearance of the pattern, or by a verbal response ("left" or "right"). The other half of the screen contained a blank field of the same space-averaged luminance. The order of presentation (left or right half of the screen) was random. An interactive staircase procedure, which was driven by the subject's responses and controlled by the computer was used. Presentation time was limited (500msec), but decision time was unlimited. An average of 20 reversals of the staircase constituted the mean value of an individual spatial frequency. The reciprocal of the spatial contrast detection threshold was used as a measure for spatial contrast sensitivity. Figure 3.1 shows contrast sensitivity profiles of a group of normal control subjects and of individual patients with unilateral or bilateral posterior brain injury. Patients may show either global reduction of contrast sensitivity or contrast sensitivity loss selective for spatial frequencies (see also Bodis-Wollner, 1972, 1976; Bodis-Wollner & Diamond,

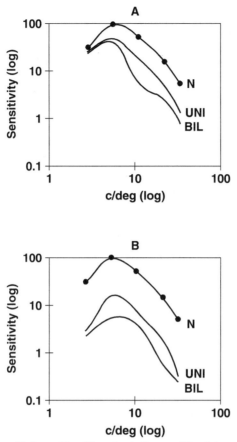

FIG. 3.1   Contrast sensitivity profiles (binocular testing conditions) in a group of five normal control subjects (N), a patient with unilateral (UNI) and bilateral (BIL) occipital stroke. A: examples for moderate, B: for severe impairment in spatial contrast sensitivity. c/deg: cycles/degree.

1976; Bulens et al., 1989; Hess et al., 1990). Patients with impaired spatial contrast sensitivity especially report difficulties with reading, because characters appear "unclear" and as "merging one into another".

Spontaneous recovery of contrast sensitivity

Bodis-Wollner (1972) reported impaired spatial contrast sensitivity in two patients who had tumours in the posterior brain. Both patients showed (spontaneous) recovery within 6–8 weeks after treatment with antibiotics (case 1), and after surgical removal and steroid medication (case 2). Although contrast sensitivity remained depressed in both cases, these observations indicate that this visual function can, in part, return. On the other hand, in the group of 62 patients with uni- or bilateral posterior brain injury reported by Hess et al. (1990), severely reduced spatial contrast sensitivity was found in patients who had suffered brain injury up to several years before testing. The outcome of this study indicates that visual contrast sensitivity can be permanently impaired.

Practice of contrast sensitivity

The report of Bodis-Wollner (1972) on spontaneous recovery of contrast sensit- ivity, and an earlier report on perceptual learning specific for spatial frequency (Fiorentini & Berardi, 1980) suggest that the specific practice of the detection of gratings might lead to better contrast sensitivity. In three cases we have tried to improve spatial contrast sensitivity by giving patients training in pattern detec- tion at the threshold level. We used the same procedure for practice and for testing, except that only three (2.8, 11.2, 33.6 c/deg) spatial frequencies were used for practice, and six spatial frequencies for the pre- and post-tests. Further- more, since two patients also showed considerably reduced visual acuity, we measured visual acuity before and after practice to assess the effect of a possibly improved spatial contrast sensitivity on visual acuity.

All three patients complained of pronounced visual blurring especially when reading. The visual environment appeared "foggy" and patients reported being considerably impaired in many of their daily activities. Two patients (P1, P2; both males; 49 and 56 years old) suffered left- (P1) and right-sided (P2) occipital infarction; the third patient (P3; female, aged 36 years) suffered bilateral occipital haemorrhage. Time since brain injury was 6 weeks in P1, 7 weeks in P2, and 9 weeks in P3. P1 and P2 showed incomplete hemianopia, with field sparing of 6° (P1) and 8° (P2). P3 suffered from bilateral hemianopia (diameter of spared visual field = 14°). Binocular visual acuity (Snellen fraction) was 1.0 in P1, 0.65 in P2, and 0.10 in P3. Since patients found the training of the detection of gratings very demanding and complained of fatigue after about 20– 30 presentations, breaks of 1–3 minutes were introduced after blocks of 25 presentations and the number of blocks was limited to 5 in a single practice session. In Fig. 3.2 the outcome of the treatment is shown. Spatial contrast sensitivity had improved, to varying degrees, in all patients. Improvement was not restricted to the spatial frequencies used for practice, but showed generalisa- tion to other frequencies. However, the improvement in all patients was most pronounced in the middle range of frequencies which are known to be especially important in vision and show the lowest thresholds in normal subjects (Sekuler & Blake, 1985). Interestingly, after practice of contrast sensitivity patients also showed higher visual acuity values. In P2 acuity returned to normal (Snellen fraction = 1.0), while P3 exhibited a partial improvement (Snellen fraction = 0.40). P1 and P2 reported a distinct improvement in "clear vision", especially con- cerning reading. Before practice with contrast sensitivity reading performance (text consisting of 180 words in 20 lines; Univers, 12 pt) was 70 wpm in P1 and

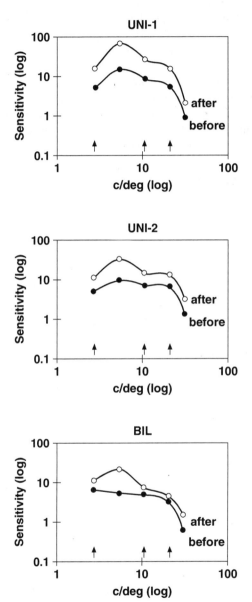

FIG. 3.2 Contrast sensitivity profiles before and after practice with spatial contrast vision in two patients (UNI-1, UNI-2) with unilateral and one patient with bilateral (BIL) occipital stroke. c/deg: cycles/degree. Arrows indicate spatial frequencies selected for practice (see text). Note the increase in sensitivity after practice especially in the medium range of spatial frequencies.

64 wpm in P2; P3 was unable to read. After practice, P1 read at a speed of 139 wpm and P2 at a speed of 121 wpm. P3 could eventually correctly read 21 out of 30 single words in larger print (Univers, 18 pt).

Our observations produce preliminary evidence that spatial contrast sensitivity can, in principle, be improved by specific and systematic practice. However, the limited number of cases does not allow definite conclusions to be drawn about who might benefit from this type of treatment and what the main effects would be in terms of reduction of visual disability. Furthermore, for methodological reasons the use of different procedures for treatment and assessment of the treatment effect would be desirable.

LIGHT AND DARK ADAPTATION

Light and dark adaptation can be affected after uni- as well as bilateral postchiasmatic brain injury (Zihl & Kerkhoff, 1990). Patients with impaired light adaptation often complain of a strong sensation of being "blinded" under normal daylight or artificial illumination conditions. They find it very unpleasant to look, for example, at a white sheet of paper because its reflection of light causes blinding and text may appear "blurred" or even fade. Patients suffering from impaired dark adaptation typically report that the surroundings appear "too dark", even under normal daylight or artificial illumination conditions. This "darkening" impairs identification of faces and objects, especially on black and white photographs, and reading. A third group of patients may suffer from impaired light and dark adaptation. This condition undoubtedly is the most problematic because normal illumination is not sufficient for "clear vision", but at the same time causes "blinding". In a study on 116 brain-injured patients, we (Zihl & Kerkhoff, 1990) found impaired visual adaptation in 90 cases (78%); 23 patients (26%) showed impaired light adaptation, 21 (23%) impaired dark adaptation, and 46 (51%) impaired light and dark adaptation. All patients reported that the symptoms mentioned were not present before the onset of brain injury, but occurred "suddenly" afterwards. Compared to normal control subjects, patients with impaired light adaptation preferred lower, while patients with impaired dark adaptation preferred higher illumination values. Patients with impaired light and dark adaptation rated illumination similarly to patients with impaired light adaptation, i.e. they also preferred lower illumination levels although this illumination was often insufficient for normal reading, for example.

Unfortunately no follow-up observations are available concerning spontaneous recovery of visual adaptation. However, time since brain injury was in the range of 2 months up to more than 6 years in our study (Zihl & Kerkhoff, 1990), suggesting that this visual disorder can persist. Patients with defective light adaptation may benefit from sunglasses and variable adjustment of illumination, especially when reading. In our experience, patients with impaired dark adaptation should always adjust illumination in rooms as much as necessary for reading or work. Patients with impaired light and dark adaptation should make use of both means. In addition, there is evidence that the use of light-filtering lenses can reduce intolerance to light in brain-injured patients. Jackowski, Sturr, Taub, and Turk (1996) reported reduction in the degree of intolerance to light and a significant enhancement of contrast sensitivity and improved reading in a group of seven patients with traumatic brain injury when provided with such lenses. Although the authors do not report details on visual adaptation or contrast sensitivity, these preliminary findings appear promising. Light-filtering lenses may thus be an appropriate means for patients who report "photophobia" after acquired brain injury.

CHAPTER FOUR

Colour vision deficits

After unilateral occipitotemporal brain injury colour vision may be lost in the contralateral hemifield or the upper quadrant (Albert, Reches, & Silverberg, 1975; Damasio et al., 1980; Henderson, 1982; Poulson, Galetta, Grossman, & Alavi, 1994; Zihl & von Cramon, 1986b). Patients are usually aware of this disorder and report that the corresponding part of the visual surroundings appears "very pale" or in "black and white", "like in an old movie". For mapping this visual field disorder, coloured instead of white targets are used (Aulhorn & Harms, 1972). It is important to note that in these cases light sensitivity and form vision are not impaired in the affected hemifield, indicating that the loss of colour vision is selective (Zihl & Mayer, 1981). Foveal colour vision may also be affected; patients typically report that fine colour hue discrimination has become difficult for them since the onset of brain injury. In our experience, professionals (e.g. painters) and female patients (possibly because they care more about colours when composing their dress or a bouquet of flowers) are more often aware of difficulties in using fine colour hues after acquired brain injury.

Impairments in colour hue discrimination can best be assessed by means of the Farnsworth–Munsell 100-hue test (FM 100-hue test; Farnsworth, 1943; Meadows, 1974; Zihl, Roth, Kerkhoff, & Heywood, 1988; Fig. 4.1). Subjects are asked to sort colour hues such that the next hue fits best to the preceding one, whereby the first and the last hue of a row are shown as "anchors".

In patients with bilateral occipitotemporal injury, colour vision may be moderately affected in the entire visual field (cerebral dyschromatopsia; Rizzo, Smith, Pokorny, & Damasio, 1993), or in rare cases may even be completely lost (cerebral achromatopsia; Damasio et al., 1980; Meadows, 1974; Pearlman, Birch,

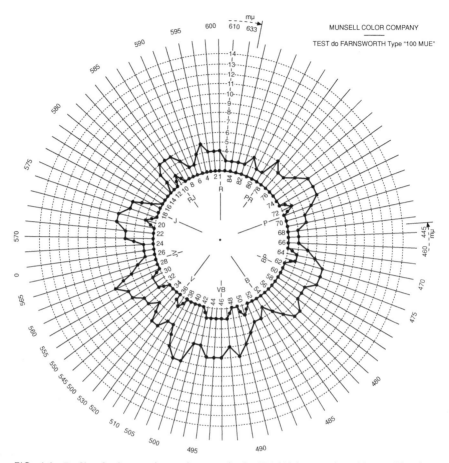

FIG. 4.1 Profile of colour sorting performance in the FM 100-hue test in a 46-year-old patient with dyschromatopsia after unilateral (left-sided) occipitotemporal stroke. Inner profile represents sorting performance of an age-matched control subject. Test scores = patient 391, normal subject = 187.

& Meadows, 1979; Pöppel et al., 1978; Zihl & von Cramon, 1986b). All capacities that involve colour may be affected: discrimination and sorting of colours, naming of colours, and association of colours with their names and with objects which have a particular colour as a characteristic feature (e.g. yellow and banana; red and strawberry; green and grass; blue and sky). In the FM 100-hue test, these patients show a considerably higher number of errors compared with patients suffering from unilateral posterior brain injury (Fig. 4.2). In contrast, greys can often be differentiated correctly (Heywood, Wilson, & Cowey, 1987). In everyday life, these patients may report that objects and pictures look "pale", are "drained of colour", have a "dirty brownish" or "reddish" appearance, or are in "black and white".

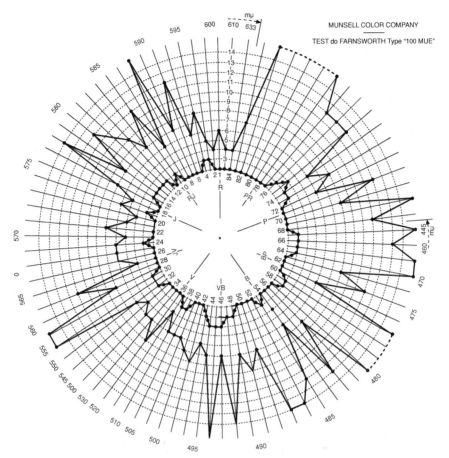

FIG. 4.2 Profile of colour sorting in FM 100-hue test in profiles in a 64-year-old patient with dyschromatopsia after bilateral occipitotemporal stroke. Inner profile represents sorting performance of an age-matched control subject. Test scores: patient = 839, normal subject = 207.

SPONTANEOUS RECOVERY

Recovery of colour vision has been observed in patients with complete cerebral blindness and spontaneous return of vision (see p. 16). In the achromatopsic case described by Pearlman et al. (1979), no spontaneous recovery was observed over a period of 6 years. Systematic follow-up studies on spontaneous recovery of colour perception or colour discrimination, or improvement after specific practice, respectively, are missing however. As already mentioned, not all patients with moderately impaired colour vision after unilateral posterior brain injury are aware of their deficit and therefore will not report it, especially if fine colour discrimination is neither essential nor important for professional or other reasons. The absence of colour vision in one hemifield is typically associated with an "unpleasant feeling", as one patient with a left-sided hemiachromatopsia described it, but does not cause a visual disability, because patients can still correctly differentiate and recognise forms and can read. They have no difficulties detecting stimuli appearing on the affected side and shifting their gaze accurately towards them. In our experience, after several weeks patients are no longer aware of these feelings and seem to have adapted to this condition. It would, of course, be very interesting to know whether in these cases some kind of a "filling in" has taken place, as is known for smaller blind field regions (see Pöppel, 1986; Sergent, 1988).

PRACTICE OF COLOUR VISION

Among 786 patients with visual disorders after acquired posterior brain injury, who were seen by us in the past 20 years, only 8 cases (< 1%) showed severely impaired colour vision, all of them after bilateral posterior brain injury. Here we report training effects in two patients with cerebral dyschromatopsia after brain injury. The first patient (P1), then a 53-year-old businessman, had lost colour vision almost completely after bilateral posterior infarction. For him, colour vision was crucial for continuing his profession. The FM 100-hue test was carried out for the first time 9 months after his stroke, which was 17 months before specific practice of colour discrimination. The second patient (P2), a 21-year-old student, in addition to visual agnosia (see pp. 136–137) had severely impaired colour vision after a traffic accident, in which he had suffered severe cerebral hypoxia after closed head injury, a condition known to cause cerebral achromatopsia (Young, Fishman, & Chen, 1980). The FM 100-hue test was carried out in this patient 16 months after brain injury, which was 10 months before specific practice. P1 could report the correct colour from memory when asked to name the colour of, for example, flowers, fruits or animals, while P2 also had difficulties with colour imagery and colour naming.

The practice method which was used to improve colour discrimination was adopted from experiments with monkeys who after experimental lesions showed impairments in hue discrimination (e.g. Heywood, Gadotti, & Cowey, 1992). Colour stimuli were generated using a specially developed software program and were presented on a high resolution screen. Room illumination was low (< 5 lux) to help prevent blinding effects on the monitor. The various hues were calibrated by means of the *Munsell Book of Color* (1976); stimulus luminance was equated so that differences between different colours were less than 2%. In the first phase of practice, patients were given pairs of colours of different categories, e.g. red and blue. In the second phase pairs of colour hues within the same category and in the third phase, triplets of colours taken from the same category were used. Differences between hues in the first and second phases were successively reduced to make discrimination more and more difficult thereby improving discrimination sensitivity. In the first two phases of practice patients were asked to tell whether the two hues were the same or different. In the third phase they were instructed to take the odd one out. It is important to note that patients never had to name the colour hues. A method of so-called errorless discrimination was used, where subjects were always reinforced for the correct response, and errors were eliminated immediately (Sidman & Stoddard, 1967). Tables 4.1A&B summarise the procedure in both patients. To assess the effect of practice, we measured colour discrimination capacity with the FM 100-hue

TABLE 4.1A

Procedure of practice with colour hue discrimination in two patients with cerebral dyschromatopsia after bilateral posterior brain injury. Hues were selected on the basis of corresponding values in the *Munsell Book of Color* (1976). Phase 1: Discrimination of two colours between different categories (same–different)

Stimuli	*Colours*
Colour stimuli	
Red	6.25R, 4/12
Green	1.25G, 5/12
Blue	5B, 4/10
Yellow	2.5Y, 8/12
Stimulus combinations	Red–Green, Red–Blue, Red–Yellow
	Green–Blue, Green–Yellow
	Blue–Yellow

TABLE 4.1B

Patients as in Table 4.1A. Phase 2: Discrimination of two colours within the same category (same–different) Phase 3: Take-the-*odd*-one-out-paradigm (2 identical hues, 1 different hue). Identical hues in Phase 3 are indicated in italics

Phase	*Red (2.5R)*	*Green (7.5GY)*	*Blue (7.5B)*	*Yellow (2.5Y)*
2	4/14–6/12	5/8–7/12	5/10–7/8	8/16–8/10
	5/14–3/10	6/10–8/12	4/10–6/8	7/12–8.5/12
	5/12–4/12	5/8–7/12	6/10–4/10	6/10–8/10
	5/14–6/10	7/10–6/8	6/6–5/8	8/12–8/8
	4/14–3/10	6/8–7/12	4/8–6/6	7/12–6/10
3	*5/12–5/10*	*5/10–5/8*	*5/10–4/10*	*7/12–8/14*
	5/14–5/12	*5/12–5/10*	*6/10–5/10*	*8/14–8/10*
	4/12–4/10	*6/10–5/10*	*5/8–4/8*	*8/12–8/8*
	4/14–4/12	*7/10–6/10*	*6/8–5/8*	*7/10–6/10*
	6/10–6/8	*7/10–6/10*	*6/8–7/8*	*8/16–8/12*
	6/12–6/10	*8/10–7/10*	*6/10–6/8*	*8/10–8/16*
	4/10–5/10	*7/8–6/10*	*4/8–4/6*	*8/12–7/12*
	3/10–4/10	*7/10–7/8*	*4/10–4/8*	*8.5/10–8/12*
	5/12–4/12	*8/8–6/10*	*6/8–6/6*	*8/8–8.5/12*
	6/12–5/12	*8/10–8/6*	*7/6–6/8*	*8/16–8/8*

test before and after treatment and in addition tested patients' naming ability for colours using coloured photographs with objects that do not possess a particular colour as a characteristic feature (e.g. cars, clothing, buildings). Patients were asked to identify the colour of the objects by naming the corresponding colour.

As can be seen in Table 4.2, both patients benefited from practice with colour discrimination. The performance for identifying the odd one out was 86% in patient 1 and 92% in patient 2, even after the distances between hues were considerably decreased in both subjects. Figures 4.3 and 4.4 show the outcome of systematic practice with colour discrimination as assessed by the FM 100-hue test. At the first time of testing P1 (9 months post-injury) had a score of 689 and P2 (16 months post-injury) a score of 605 in this test. For comparison, the corresponding values for age-matched normal subjects were 202 and 176, respectively. Before treatment, i.e. 26 months after brain injury in P1 and P2, the corresponding scores were 682 and 611. After treatment, both patients showed a considerably better discrimination performance; the scores were now 361 in P1

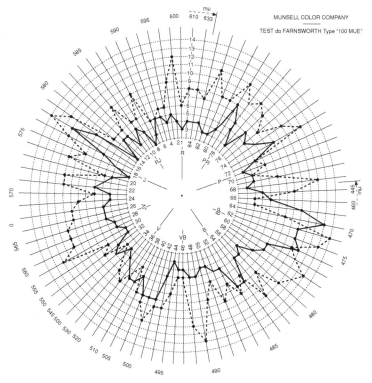

FIG. 4.3   Colour sorting performance in the FM 100-hue test before (broken lines) and after (solid lines) practice with colour discrimination in a patient (P1) with bilateral occipitotemporal stroke. Test scores: before practice = 611, after practice = 378.

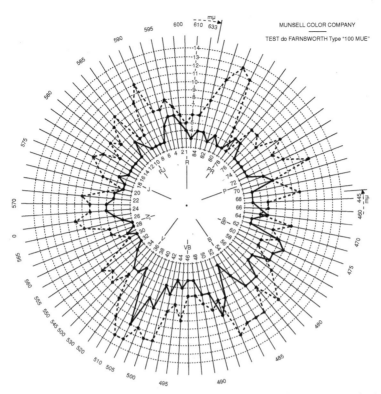

FIG. 4.4 Effect of practice with colour discrimination on colour sorting performance in the FM 100-hue test before (broken lines) and after (solid lines) practice in a patient (P2) with cerebral hypoxia. Test scores: before practice = 682, after practice = 361.

TABLE 4.2

Improvement in colour discrimination in two patients (P1, P2) with cerebral dyschromatopsia in same–different judgements between (A) and within (B) categories, and in a take-the-odd-one-out paradigm (C) (see Table 4.1)

			Red		Green		Blue		Yellow	
	No. of trials	No. of sessions	Before % correct	After	Before % correct	After	Before % correct	After	Before % correct	After
(A)										
P1	600	6	80	92	64	72	56	72	64	88
P2	600	6	58	92	24	64	20	60	36	82
(B)										
P1	760	5	70	88	40	70	33	78	55	80
P2	900	5	47	82	27	69	36	58	40	80
(C)										
P1	1200	10	68	89	53	70	60	75	65	83
P2	1600	10	73	93	48	70	43	65	53	85

$n = 40$ trials/category.

105

and 378 in P2. Thus, the main improvement occurred during the period of training of colour discrimination. The improvement in colour discrimination also became evident in the recognition of coloured objects and in colour naming (Table 4.3). Since colour naming was not trained in either patient, this result may be taken as evidence that the difficulty with colour naming at least in P1 was mainly due to impaired colour perception.

Both patients benefited from the improvement in colour vision. P1 reported being able once again to compare and select, at least in part, colour hues on textiles. P2 could use colours for better identification of objects (see p. 41).

Taken together, these observations suggest that impaired colour vision in brain-injured patients can be improved by systematic practice. Although our approach was mainly of experimental character, the outcome may hopefully stimulate further attempts to remediate colour vision deficiency after acquired brain injury.

TABLE 4.3

Naming of colours before and after practice with colour discrimination in two patients with cerebral dyschromatopsia

	Red		Green		Blue		Yellow	
	Before	After	Before	After	Before	After	Before	After
	% correct		% correct		% correct		% correct	
P1	56	96	48	88	50	88	54	94
P2	48	88	24	74	26	66	42	92

$n = 25$ trials per hue.

CHAPTER FIVE

Disorders in visual space perception

Disorders in visual space perception comprise various impairments, ranging from elementary deficits, for example visual localisation, up to complex disorders such as spatial cognition and visuoconstructive abilities. Such disorders are typically observed after occipitoparietal injury, with a right-hemisphere injury more frequently causing deficits in "higher" visual spatial capacities (for comprehensive reviews, see Benton & Tranel, 1993; De Renzi, 1982; Grüsser & Landis, 1991).

In patients with unilateral brain injury, defective visual spatial localisation is typically observed in the hemifield contralateral to the side of brain injury. Although this impairment may affect saccadic localisation accuracy (Fig. 5.1 and Table 5.1), patients usually do not complain of difficulties with visual spatial localisation in everyday life activities. In contrast, patients with bilateral posterior brain injury with disturbance of saccadic localisation in the entire visual field, typically report moderate to severe difficulties in visually guided activities (see Figs. 5.1 and 5.2). These activities especially concern the accurate fixation of objects, reading and writing, and reaching for objects.

A further visual spatial deficit concerns a systematic shift in the vertical and horizontal axes and the egocentric visual midline opposite to the side of brain injury (Table 5.2). Shifts in the vertical and horizontal axes have especially been observed in patients with right occipitoparietal injury (Kerkhoff, 1988; Lütgehetmann & Stäbler, 1992). Shifts in the straight-ahead direction have been reported in patients with left- and right-sided occipital and occipitoparietal injury. They are frequently associated with homonymous visual field defects, but are not caused by them, because no systematic relationship has been found between the degree of visual field sparing and the deviation from the objective

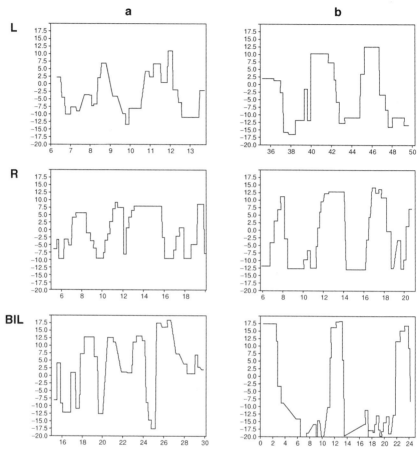

FIG. 5.1 Saccadic localisation (voluntary horizontal eye movements) in patients with left (L), right (R), and bilateral (BIL) posterior parietal injury without field defects to targets in the left and right hemifield. a: 20° distance, b: 30° distance. Bottom: left, top: right. x-axis: time period of recording (in seconds); y-axis: horizontal amplitude (in degrees) of saccades (0 = centre). Note saccadic dysmetria (hypo- and hypermetria) in all cases to both sides. For corresponding eye movement recordings in normal control subjects, see Fig. 2.7.

TABLE 5.1

Saccadic accuracy for horizontal target positions in patients with unilateral (left, right) and with bilateral posterior brain injury

	Direction of eye movement	20° (n = 20) M (1SD)	30° (n = 20) M (1SD)
Left (n = 5)	←	8.1° (2.5)	8.9° (3.6)
	→	11.9° (4.3)	17.0° (6.8)
Right (n = 5)	←	11.0° (3.1)	17.1° (7.7)
	→	13.4° (5.2)	14.7° (7.3)
Bilateral (n = 5)	←	9.1° (4.8)	8.9° (5.2)
	→	9.9° (6.7)	10.5° (6.8)

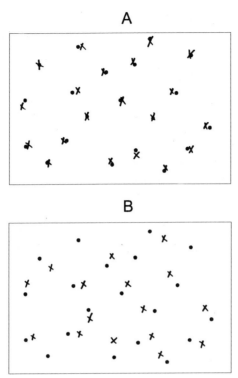

FIG. 5.2 Dot cancellation in a patient with unilateral (right-sided) (A) and with bilateral posterior parietal injury (B). Note moderate inaccuracy of crossing out responses in A and pronounced inaccuracy in B.

TABLE 5.2
Shift in the straight-ahead direction in 10 patients with left-sided (LH)
and 10 with right-sided (RH) hemianopia

Patient	LH: VFSP (°)	Shift (° visual angle)	RH: VFSP (°)	Shift (° visual angle)
1	1	2.9	1	4.6
2	1	3.8	1	3.8
3	1	3.1	1	3.8
4	2	2.3	2	6.0
5	2	2.5	2	2.3
6	2	5.3	3	2.8
7	3	4.8	4	3.8
8	3	2.7	4	3.4
9	4	3.6	4	3.1
10	4	3.1	5	2.9
Mean (1SD)	2.3 (1.2)	3.3 (0.9)	2.7 (1.5)	3.4 (1.2)

VFSP: visual field sparing. All LH-patients shifted to the left, all RH-patients to the right side.

centre (Zihl & von Cramon, 1986b; see Table 5.2). However, because of the frequent association, Liepman and Kalmus, who first described this visual disorder in 1900, coined the term "hemianopic measurement error". As a consequence of these shifts in the visual vertical and horizontal axes, patients may have difficulty maintaining a line, for example, in writing, drawing, and copying. Patients with a shift of the egocentric visual midline have difficulties keeping the straight-ahead direction in walking along a corridor or through an entrance, or in guiding a wheelchair.

Defective depth perception and stereopsis have been reported in patients suffering from uni- and bilateral posterior brain injury, with unilateral injury causing more moderate deficits. Impaired depth perception may cause difficulties walking downstairs and reaching for objects or handles.

Finally, visual–spatial disorientation, which is often associated with hemianopia (see p. 60) and is found in its severest form in patients with the so-called Balint's syndrome (see p. 122), is also understood as a disorder of visual space perception.

SPONTANEOUS RECOVERY

Spontaneous recovery of perception of visual spatial axes has been reported by Meerwaldt (1983) within 6 months in a group of 17 patients who had suffered right posterior brain injury. In an earlier study (Meerwaldt & van Harskamp, 1982) on the recovery from visual spatial deficits after right posterior brain injury, only a slight improvement was found. Hier et al. (1983b) reported recovery from visuospatial and visuoconstructive deficits in 70% of 41 patients within about 4 months after stroke. Unfortunately, no information is available regarding the behavioural significance of the observed improvements in visuospatial tests.

PRACTICE OF VISUAL LOCALISATION

Several attempts have been made to improve visual spatial abilities in brain-injured patients by means of systematic training. Diller and colleagues (Diller et al., 1974) gave their patients intensive practice in the block-design and found improvement in this task as well as increased independence in everyday life. A group of patients who participated in "standard rehabilitation" measures did not show the same degree of improvement. Weinberg et al. (1979) trained 30 patients with right-hemisphere injury in the estimation of distances and lengths and in "sensory awareness". After 4 weeks of systematic practice, this group showed significantly higher scores on a variety of tests compared with a control group of patients who underwent "standard rehabilitation". Assessment of practice effects included reading, calculation, copying, line bisection, but also picture completion, face matching, and digit span. The outcome of these studies suggests an unspecific rather than a specific treatment effect, but the systematic occupation with visual spatial tasks undoubtedly also had beneficial effects on visual–spatial abilities. It appears very likely, however, that the poor performance before treatment was mainly due to the visual neglect which not only affected visual–spatial capacities, but all tasks involving operations in space, including shifting of attention and of fixation. One may hypothesise, therefore, that the observed improvements in visual tests as well as in activities of daily living (ADL) scores can be explained by the recovery from visual neglect and by the improved attentional capacities and increased awareness, and not so much by the "specific rehabilitation" of visual–spatial abilities. Kerkhoff (1988) and Lütgehetmann and Stäbler (1992) used a PC-based training programme to improve the adjustment of the visual vertical and horizontal axes, visual localisation of stimulus positions, discrimination of the length of lines, line bisection, and line orientation. At least in single cases (without visual neglect), they found significant specific improvements in performance in the various tests. Unfortunately, no evidence is presented that the improvement in the visual–spatial tests was of behavioural significance for patients.

In the following section, the effects of practice of visual spatial localisation in one patient are reported. This patient's pronounced deficits in visual spatial localisation as well as in visual spatial orientation, which also impaired object vision, reading, etc., represented a severe visual handicap in her everyday life. The patient, a 48-year-old businesswoman, had suffered bilateral occipitoparietal haemorrhage 7 months before she was first examined. She also showed incomplete amblyopia in both lower quadrants (sparing of colour and form vision along the vertical axis was 18°), reduced visual acuity (10% form acuity; see Table 5.5, p. 117), absence of stereopsis, and impaired depth perception. Colour perception was intact. Visual fixation and saccadic localisation were highly inaccurate, and she had great difficulties scanning even a simple dot stimulus array (Fig. 5.3). However, she showed no obvious signs of visual neglect or Balint's syndrome. She also had severe difficulties with visually guided reaching, with an average error of about 5°. Visual recognition was preserved, but because the patient had severe difficulties in finding objects in space and in fixating them, she showed difficulties in identifying and recognising forms, objects, and scenes. This might explain her low visual acuity when tested first time. No obvious further neurological and neuropsychological symptoms or deficits were present at the time of testing except for a paresis of the right arm and hand. In tests requiring motor responses, she therefore used her left hand.

Table 5.3 shows the training and testing procedures. We started improving the accuracy of fixation and shifting fixation as accurately as possible between two or three large (2.1° in diameter at a viewing distance of 40cm) coloured circular stimuli located 10°, 20°, or 30° apart on a white table, which she then had to touch with the index finger of her left hand. The patient was instructed to guide her eyes in such a way that she would have the "best" impression possible when fixating the stimulus, and was asked to avoid trying to control for accuracy of fixation or eye shifting by using purely "cognitive" strategies of guessing. For

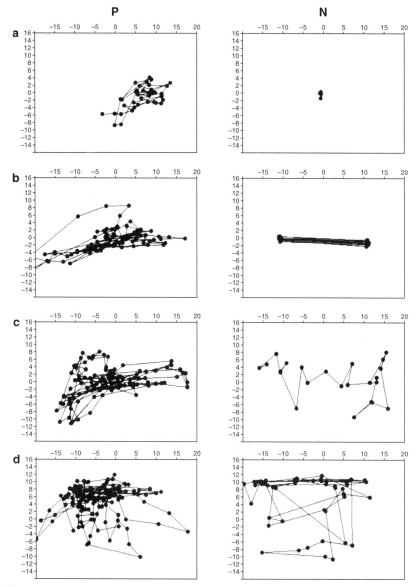

FIG. 5.3 Fixation (a; centre), voluntary saccadic eye movements (b; target distance: 20°), scanning of a dot pattern (Fig. 2.6B; c), and scanning of a scene (d; 7 items: 6 fishermen and a dog; see Fig. 6.1) in a patient with bilateral posterior parietal brain injury (P) and in an age-matched normal subject (N). Recording time in (a) was 30sec for P and 15sec for N; in (b) it was 60sec for P and 30sec for N. Scanning times in (c) and (d) were 64.7 and 75.7sec for P, and 8.3 and 16.0sec for N. The patient reported only 11 out of 20 dots in (c) and 3 out of 7 items in (d); the normal control subject reported correctly all items in both tasks. Note the highly inaccurate fixation of the patient in (a) and (b) and the lack of spatial organisation of oculomotor scanning in (c) and (d). x-axis: horizontal extension of stimulus array (in degrees; 0 = centre, negative values left, positive values right), y-axis: vertical extension (0 = centre, negative values down, positive values up). Dots indicate fixation locations. For further details, see Fig. 5.1.

TABLE 5.3
Plan of treatment in a patient with severe visual spatial deficits
after bilateral posterior parietal injury

Phase	Treatment
1	*Localisation of single visual objects by fixating and reaching* 2–3 Objects; spatial separations: 10°, 20°, and 30° 2640 trials in 22 sessions
2	*Saccadic localisation of visual targets in the perimeter* 1–3 positions in the left and right hemifields at 10°, 20°, and 30° 3600 trials in 20 sessions
3	*Visual search on slides and on a monitor* Slides: 1560 presentations in 26 sessions Monitor: 2496 presentations in 22 sessions
4	*Touching* Localisation of 2–6 positions on a touch screen 1890 trials in 21 sessions
5	*Reading* Tachistoscopic presentation of single words 1620 presentations in 9 sessions

the feedback for fixation accuracy she was asked to use her "best vision" of the stimulus. After 2420 trials in 18 sessions a fairly good performance in fixation accuracy and in shifting fixation between stimulus positions was obtained. The Tübingen perimeter was then used to improve saccadic localisation for a wider range of distances along the left and right horizontal axes.

The procedure was identical to that described earlier for enlarging saccadic movements (p. 37), except that we started with only one target position in each hemifield and later increased the number of positions up to three in each field. Presentation time was 5–7sec at the beginning and was later reduced to 1sec or even 500msec. In nine sessions 3600 trials of practice were carried out. As Fig. 5.4 shows, the patient could not only fixate a target and shift fixation more accurately after practice; her scanning behaviour was also improved. Finally, we gave the patient practice in visual scanning and visual search in the slide and the monitor conditions (see pp. 48 and 61). A further improvement was found after this type of practice (Fig. 5.5 and Table 5.4). She now also reported an improvement in vision in her everyday life. For example, she was again able to reach accurately for the door handle, to pick up food accurately with the fork, and to put on make-up using a mirror. The improved accuracy in fixation may well also have enabled the patient to fixate objects more accurately and therefore to have less difficulty localising and identifying them, and also reaching for them. We therefore reassessed visual acuity and visual recognition at this stage and found considerable improvement for both visual abilities (Table 5.5).

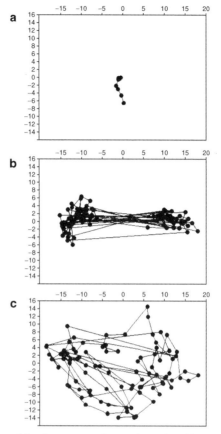

FIG. 5.4 Improvement of fixation accuracy in a patient with bilateral posterior parietal injury (same patient as in Fig. 5.3) after practice with visual localisation: fixation in the centre (a; 30sec), voluntary saccadic eye movements (b; 60sec), and scanning of the dot pattern (c; scanning time: 46.6sec). The patient now reported 13 out 20 dots. Further details as in Figs. 5.1 and 5.3.

In the next stage, we gave the patient specific practice in reaching for a visual target by using a touch screen. Unfortunately, we could not measure her ability to touch targets at the very beginning of treatment. We do not know therefore whether the patient had already benefited from the systematic practice of saccadic localisation. For testing her reaching accuracy, we developed a software program to generate and present targets on a touch screen, on which positions, number of targets, and presentation time could be varied. The patient sat at a distance of 50cm in front of the screen; at this distance, the screen subtended 38.7° horizontally, and 31° vertically. Target diameter was 1.1°; targets were shown in yellow on a black background. Room illumination was low (1 lux) to help prevent blinding and cueing effects on the monitor. A trial was started with the presentation of a blue cross in the centre of the screen which disappeared with the onset of target presentation. The patient was asked to fixate the blue

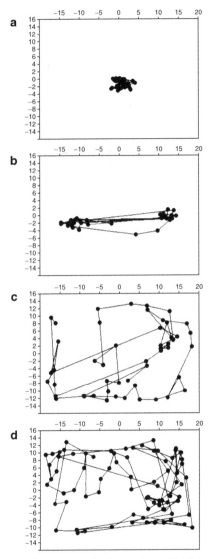

FIG. 5.5 Improvement of oculomotor scanning in a patient with bilateral posterior parietal injury (same patient as in Fig. 5.3) after practice with visual search. Stimulus conditions as in Fig. 5.3. a: Fixation in the centre (30sec); b: voluntary saccadic eye movements (30sec), c: scanning of the dot pattern (scanning time: 31.6sec), d: scanning of a scene (41.4sec). The patient reported 16 out of 20 dots in (c), and 5 out of 7 items in (d). Further details as in Figs. 5.1 and 5.3.

cross, and when a single target appeared to touch it as accurately as possible with the index finger of her left hand. We started with the central position and then used two and later four stimulus positions. Stimuli appeared at random and did not disappear until the patient had touched the respective position.

TABLE 5.4

Eye movement parameters in a patient with severe visual spatial deficits after bilateral posterior parietal injury at different stages of practice (for description of training phases, see Table 5.3)

Eye movement parameter	Phase M (ISD)				FIX	FIXr (%)	FD (sec) M (ISD)	A (°) M (ISD)
	1	2	3	4				
Fixation accuracy (deviation)								
P	3.6° (1.7)	2.1° (1.5)	2.2° (1.4)	1.8° (1.2)				
N	1.2° (0.6)			1.1° (0.8)				
Saccadic accuracy								
P	4.2° (1.3)	7.3° (1.7)	12.6° (2.6)	13.3° (3.2)				
N	20.9° (1.1)			19.8° (1.4)				
Scanning: dot pattern								
P Phase 1					144	62.5	0.36 (0.12)	3.7 (1.3)
Phase 2					93	35.5	0.32 (0.09)	4.7 (1.8)
Phase 3					50	24.0	0.28 (0.06)	5.3 (2.9)
Phase 4					44	26.0	0.26 (0.07)	5.5 (3.1)
N					23	13.0	0.22 (0.05)	5.8 (2.4)
Scanning: scene								
P Phase 1					110	54.5	0.38 (0.14)	4.2 (1.6)
Phase 4					80	26.2	0.28 (0.08)	5.3 (2.7)
N					48	23.8	0.24 (0.09)	6.7 (2.9)

Saccadic accuracy: localisation of targets separated by 20°. FIX: number of fixations, FIXr: percentage of repetitions of fixations, FD: fixation duration, A: saccadic amplitudes. Fixation was recorded during 30 sec; 20 saccades were performed to either side. Corresponding values of an age-matched normal subject are shown for comparison (cf. Fig. 5.3). P: patient, N: normal subject.

TABLE 5.5

Visual acuity (binocular form acuity; Snellen fractions; means of 5 measurements; (A) and visual identification of objects and scenes ($n = 30$); (B) in a patient with severe visual spatial deficits after bilateral posterior parietal injury at different stages of treatment. For description of training phases, see Table 5.3

	Form	Snellen	Objects (%)	Scenes (%)
(A) Acuity				
Before training	0.10	–		
After phase 1	0.40	0.13		
After phase 2	0.60	0.22		
After phase 3	0.70	0.29		
After phase 4	0.80	0.30		
(B) Visual identification				
Before training			40	20
After training			80	53

After about 300 trials for each position (a total of 1800 trials), we found considerable improvement, but the patient was still unable to touch the target with high accuracy (see Figs. 5.6 and 5.7). Nevertheless, when accuracy of visual reaching for objects was compared before and after training, the patient performed much better. This observed improvement is paralleled by the outcome of a dot cancellation task (Fig. 5.8), where the patient showed less difficulties after practice. She reported a distinct improvement in reaching for objects in her everyday life. For example, she could now reach accurately for a glass of wine or a cup of tea. Certainly, natural objects contain more visual cues that can be used for visually guided reaching (and of course grasping) than light targets on a screen; nevertheless the patient benefited from practice in this artificial condition at least to some degree.

Finally, we examined reading, aware of the fact that reading requires a highly accurate visual guidance of eye movements. Figure 5.9 shows recordings of eye movements during reading (for recording conditions, see p. 22). Even after intensive practice in spatial visual tasks, the patient was still unable to read, although she could correctly decipher single words consisting of three to four characters. For a more specific practice of reading, we used tachistoscopic presentation of words (see p. 81), starting with very short words (two to three characters). Table 5.6 shows reading performance for each block of text material and the number of sessions. After practice, the patient required less time to read correctly even longer words, and could now also read short sentences, but reading of "normal" text was still impossible. Nevertheless she was quite happy about this improvement, because it enabled her "at least to know that reading will be possible again".

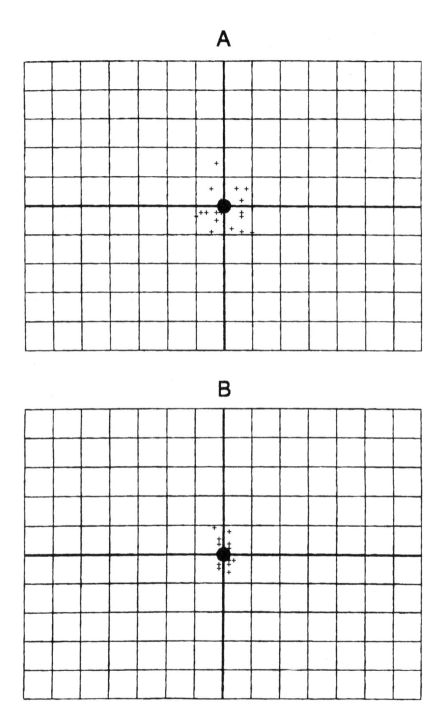

A

B

FIG. 5.6   Touch performance (one-target-condition) before (A) and after (B) practice in a patient with bilateral posterior parietal injury (same patients as in Fig. 5.3). Dot: target position, crosses: patient's responses. Note improvement in touching accuracy after practice.

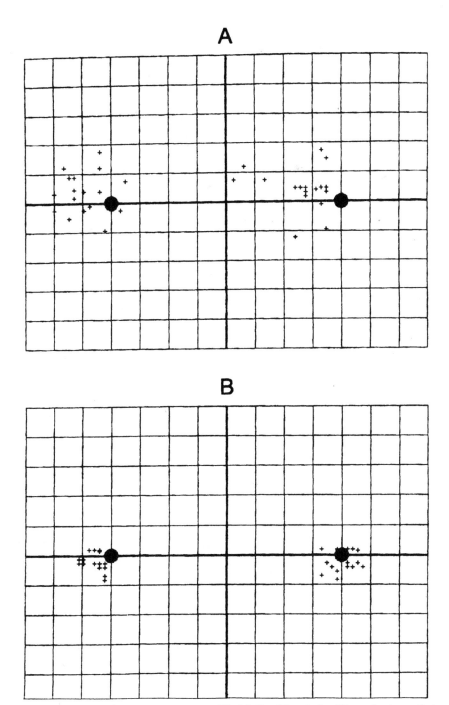

FIG. 5.7   Touch performance (two-target-condition) before (A) and after (B) practice in a patient with bilateral posterior parietal injury (same patient as in Fig. 5.3). Dots: target positions, crosses: patient's responses. Note improvement in touching accuracy after practice.

A

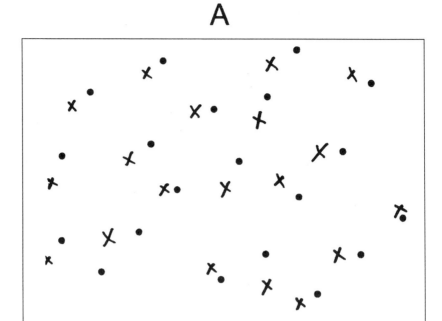

B

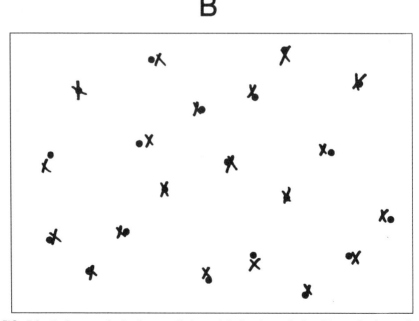

FIG. 5.8   Performance in the dot cancellation task before (A) and after (B) practice in a patient with bilateral posterior parietal injury (same patient as in Fig. 5.3). Note improved accuracy in crossing out after practice.

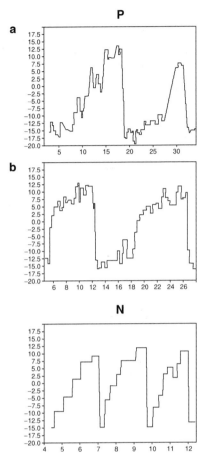

FIG. 5.9 Reading eye movements in a patient (P) with bilateral posterior parietal injury (same patient as in Fig. 5.3) before (a) and after (b) practice, and for comparison in an age-matched normal subject (N). Although the eye movement patterns still did not show the typical sequence of fixations and saccadic steps as in the normal subject, the patient was able to read singe words after practice. x-axis: time period of recording (in seconds), y-axis: horizontal extension of line (in degrees). 0 = centre, negative values left, positive values right.

In conclusion, severe visual–spatial deficits undoubtedly make great demands on rehabilitation, but, provided that appropriate methods are available, there is a good chance of reducing patients' visual disabilities by improving visual–spatial localisation and visual–spatial orientation. Although the data presented here can only serve as a hint as to how one could proceed, they may offer some helpful insight. First, a detailed analysis of a patient's "lower" and "higher" visual spatial capacities and deficits is essential for the understanding of individual visual difficulties. Second, the improvement in visual–spatial localisation of

TABLE 5.6

Practice with reading using tachistoscopic presentation in a patient with severe visual spatial deficits after bilateral posterior parietal injury

	Training procedures		Results (n = 30)	
	Presentation time (msec)	No. of trials	Before treatment (%)	After treatment (%)
2–3 letter words	2000	620		
	1000	460		
	500	320	36.7	93.3
4–5 letter words	3000	960		
	1500	920		
	750	780	20.0	90.0
3-word sentences			–	73.3

single targets also comprises visually guided fixation and reaching, but does not necessarily lead to a better visual–spatial orientation. Visual–spatial orientation appears to be a more complex capacity, involving a systematic, i.e. reliable and organised overview and coherent spatiotemporal processing, and visual–spatial working memory. Finally, reading requires its own specific spatiotemporal guidance of eye movements for coherent text information processing. Visual–spatial localisation, visual orientation, and visual–spatial guidance of reading eye movements may therefore be understood as distinct abilities with their own functional organisation, despite being based on common underlying brain mechanisms.

BALINT'S SYNDROME AND ITS TREATMENT

The term "Balint's syndrome" (named after Balint, 1909) comprises a combination of several visual symptoms, among them severe spatial (and possibly temporal) restriction of the field of visual attention and thus visual perception, impaired or even lost visual–spatial localisation and orientation, and defective depth perception (Grüsser & Landis, 1991; Pierrot-Deseilligny, Gray, & Brunet, 1986). As a consequence, patients with this syndrome can only "see" within the central portion of their visual field and are unable to see more than one or two objects or object features at a time ("simultanagnosia"). Spontaneous saccades may be absent or are at least reduced in number. On verbal command, saccades may be elicited in some cases but not in others. Patients experience great difficulties in initiating gaze shifts and in guiding their gaze from one location in space to another ("psychic paralysis of gaze"). Saccadic eye shifts are characterised by a pattern of erratic, sometimes wandering eye movements, without intentional control and correspondence to the spatial configuration of a scene or stimulus array ("oculomotor apraxia"). It becomes evident from this description that patients suffering from Balint's syndrome as a rule exhibit severe visual disabilities in their everyday lives, but also minor forms of this syndrome exist (Hecaen & Ajuriaguerra, 1954). Patients with Balint's syndrome are not very frequent; among 241 cases, Gloning, Gloning, and Hoff (1968) found only five patients (2%) with this syndrome. The underlying cause is bilateral injury to parieto-occipital structures, including occipitofrontal and parietofrontal fibre connections (Alexander & Albert, 1983).

Figure 5.10 shows examples of oculomotor scanning behaviour in two patients with Balint's syndrome. In both patients, accuracy of fixation and of saccadic localisation is highly impaired. The scanning pattern during the inspection of a dot pattern or a scene is limited to a restricted portion of the stimulus field; reading eye movements are completely absent.

Allison, Hurwitz, White, and Wilmot (1969) reported a patient with a minor form of Balint's syndrome, who after about 4 years showed good (spontaneous) recovery concerning the use of foveal vision, oculomotor scanning behaviour (fixation, saccadic eye movements), and visual–spatial orientation. In contrast to these improved capacities, reading and simultaneous perception of several objects or object features remained impaired. Montero et al. (1982) described recovery in four cases with Balint's syndrome. Three patients showed good recovery within 9–12 weeks, while in one patient vision improved slowly over a period of 5 years.

As with other "complex" but less frequent visual disorders after acquired brain injury, no study has yet been conducted on the treatment of patients with Balint's syndrome. We have tried to treat three patients (P1, P2, and P3) with severe Balint's syndrome resulting from bilateral stroke. P1 and P2 were males, P3 was female. Their ages were 58, 59, and 61 years, respectively. Time since brain injury and the beginning of treatment was 17 weeks in P1, 9 weeks in P2, and 21 weeks in P3. Accurate quantitative perimetry could not be carried out before the end of the training period. Then P1 and P3 showed bilateral hemianopia (diameter of spared field was 34° and 46°, respectively); P2 had a left-sided hemianopia (field sparing was 2°) and a right-sided hemiamblyopia (sparing of form and colour vision was 6°). In their everyday lives they were severely handicapped because of these visual disabilities. They could not find their way, the food on the plate in front of them, objects lying in front of them, etc. Thus, they needed to be treated and assisted like blind individuals.

The rationale of the treatment was to improve oculomotor functions involved in visual perception (saccadic localisation and fixation of objects), to enlarge the field of attention and to re-establish visual–spatial orientation. Except for the enlargement of the field of attention, the procedures were similar to those used to improve visual–spatial capacities described in the first part of this section (see p. 110). All patients had severe difficulties in visually guiding their eye movements, and in getting a sufficient view over words, objects, faces, and scenes. Furthermore, they never knew or were never aware of what they actually fixated,

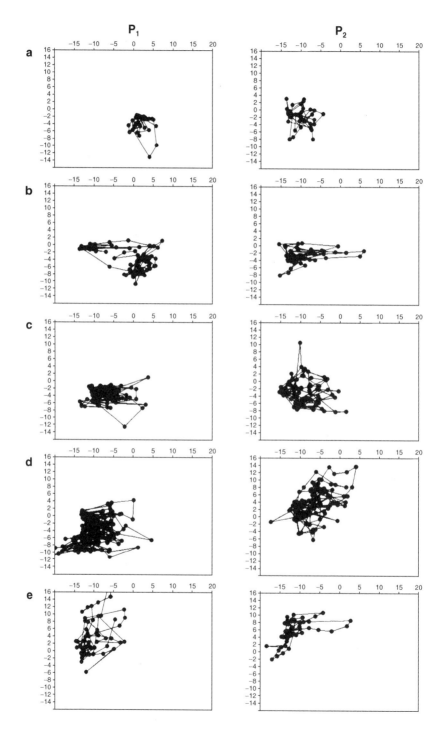

TABLE 5.7
Plan of treatment in patients with Balint's syndrome

Phase	Treatment
1	*Localisation of single visual objects by fixating and grasping* 1–3 objects; spatial separations: 5°, 10°, and 15° Stimulus field diameter: 15° –30° –45°
2	*Saccadic localisation of visual targets in the perimeter* 1–3 positions in the left and right hemifields at 10°, 20°, and 30°
3	*Visual search on slides and on a monitor* Slides: 3–15 targets (without distractors) Monitor: 1 target among 3–7 distractors

and whether they had shifted their gaze, either voluntarily or on command, to a visual stimulus or not. They always reported just one piece of a complex visual stimulus, and did not search for further information. Their visual acuity was poor, as was their form vision, and their visual recognition. However, when the acuity stimulus was brought into their small field of view, then all three patients could recognise even small forms. Under this testing condition P1 had a visual acuity of 0.8, P2 and P3 of 1.0 (Snellen fractions; binocular values). Colour vision was preserved in all patients.

Intensive practice in saccadic localisation, touching, and scanning of visual displays was given to every patient; between three and four sessions with 8–10 blocks each consisting of 10–15 trials were carried out per day. Because all patients found the training quite tiring, a break of about 3–5 minutes was introduced after each block. One session lasted about 45 minutes; the number of trials per day varied between 240 and 600. Table 5.7 shows the plan of treatment.

For the improvement of saccadic accuracy we used red, yellow, green, and blue circles (diameter = 3cm) as targets and put them one by one but at different positions within a stimulus field of 15cm in diameter in front of the patient. Before starting a practice block, patients were made familiar with the spatial extent of the area within which stimuli were shown. The idea was to give patients cues about the actual visual surroundings where they should then move

FIG. 5.10 (opposite) Fixation (a; centre), voluntary saccadic eye movements (b; target distance: 20°), scanning of a dot pattern (Fig. 2.6; c), scanning of a scene (d; 6 fishermen and a dog, cf. Fig. 6.1), and reading of one line of text (e; 6 words) in two patients with Balint's syndrome. Recording time in (a) and (b) was 60sec. Scanning times (in seconds): P1: c: 84.6, d: 116.5, e: 78.4; P2: c: 59.3; d: 59.7; e: 78.4. P1 reported 11 out of 20 dots in (c) and 3 out of 7 items in (d); P2 reported 14 dots in (c) and 2 items in (d). Note the highly inaccurate fixation of both patients in (a) and the difficulty to shift the eyes to the left and right in (b). Furthermore, the scanning patterns of both patients are severely restricted in all other stimulus conditions. For further details, see Figs. 5.1 and 5.3.

their eyes, search for the target, find it, and touch it. Touching was not to occur before the patient had found out by vision where the target was located; searching for the target by touching alone was not allowed. Between 980 (P3) and 1480 (P2) trials were carried out in this condition, with positions and colours varying at random. The therapist observed the patient's eye and hand movements carefully and gave feedback on "good" or "bad" (i.e. erroneous) eye shifts and subsequent fixation, and touch responses. After a patient showed improved visual–spatial localisation in this condition, two and later up to five targets differing in colour were presented simultaneously. Patients were told how many targets were present; before touching them they should fixate them as accurately as possible. Feedback was identical to that given in the first part of this type of practice, except that patients were forced to first glance over the area and have a global view over it, and not to search for a particular position (where they thought a target could be). The diameter of the stimulus field was now increased stepwise from 15 to 45cm. In the next phase of treatment patients were given practice with saccadic localisation of targets in the Tübingen perimeter, again starting with just one position in either hemifield and quite a long presentation time (5–8 sec). The number of positions was then continuously increased up to three in each hemifield, and presentation time was stepwise reduced to 2sec. The total number of trials in this training condition varied between 720 (P1) and 1120 (P2). Finally, patients were asked to search for targets presented on slides or an a monitor (see pp. 48 and 61). In this task, patient 1 performed 1720 trials, P2 1440, and P3 2240. In the subsequent visual search paradigm 1200 trials were carried out with P1, 1560 with P2, and 1620 with P3. Figures 5.11–5.13 show eye movement recordings for the 3 patients before and after treatment. Despite considerable differences between patients, saccadic accuracy and fixation were found to be markedly improved when compared with the recordings before practice. This finding is also underlined by the result of quantitative analysis of the recordings. Mean variability of fixation responses decreased from about 4° before practice to about 1° after practice. In addition, saccadic accuracy was found to be increased, but still very low (Table 5.8). The field of oculomotor scanning was found to be considerably enlarged after training, but all patients still exhibited signs of visual disorientation, at least in the dot pattern condition. Scanning times were longer in all patients (see Figs. 5.11–5.13 and Table 5.9), indicating that after practice patients scanned the stimulus array more carefully and within a larger area than before. After treatment, patients also showed an improved visual recognition performance for objects and scenes (Table 5.10). This improvement can best be explained by the enlargement of the field of perception and attention. The better overview now enabled the patients to use their spared visual identification and recognition abilities more efficiently. Reading, however, was still impossible after training, although patients could now decipher single words. With one patient (P2) we tried to improve reading, using a similar paradigm as in the patient with severe visual space perception

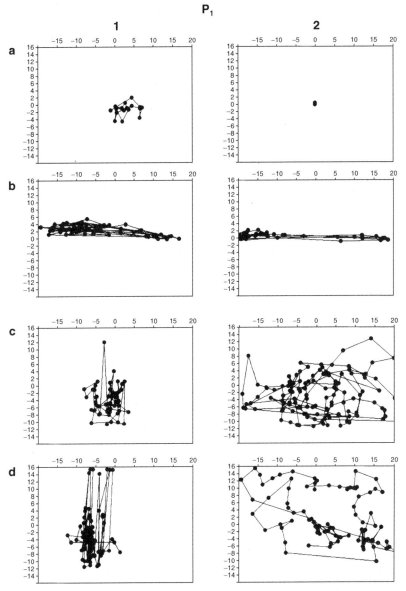

FIG. 5.11 Fixation (a; centre), voluntary saccadic eye movements (b; target distance: 20°), scanning of a dot pattern (Fig. 2.6; c), and scanning of a scene (d; 6 fishermen and a dog, cf. Fig. 6.1), in a patient with Balint's syndrome (P1; see text) before (1) and after (2) practice. Recording time in (a) and (b) was 30sec. Scanning times (in seconds): 1: c: 60.3, 2: c: 84.3; 1: d: 61.2, 2: d: 100.9. Before practice, the patient reported 11 out of 20 dots in (c) and 3 out of 7 items in (d); after practice he reported 15 dots and 5 items, respectively. Note the improvement in fixation accuracy in (2a) and (2b), and the "widening" of the field of oculomotor scanning in (2c) and (2d), which was associated with an increase in scanning time. For further description, see Figs. 5.1 and 5.3.

127

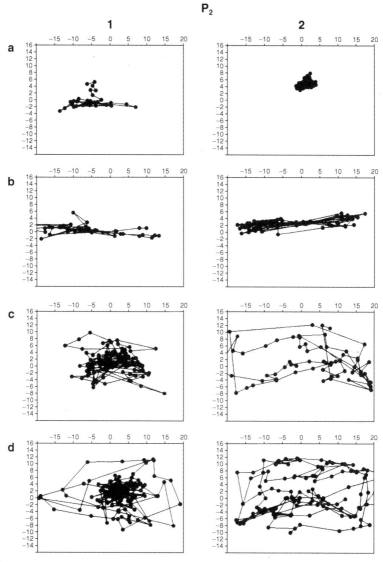

FIG. 5.12 Fixation (a; centre), voluntary saccadic eye movements (b; target distance: 20°), scanning of a dot pattern (Fig. 2.6; c), and scanning of a scene (d; 6 fishermen and a dog) in a patient with Balint's syndrome (P2; see text) before (1) and after (2) practice. Recording time in (a) and (b) was 30sec. Scanning times (in seconds): 1: c: 44.8, 2: c: 90.8; 1: d: 60.3, 2: d: 60.4. Before practice, the patient reported 12 out of 20 dots in (c) and 3 out of 7 items in (d). After practice she reported 17 dots and 5 items, respectively. Note the improvement in fixation accuracy in (2a) and (2b), and the "widening" of the field of oculomotor scanning in (2c) and (2d). For further details, see Figs. 5.1 and 5.3.

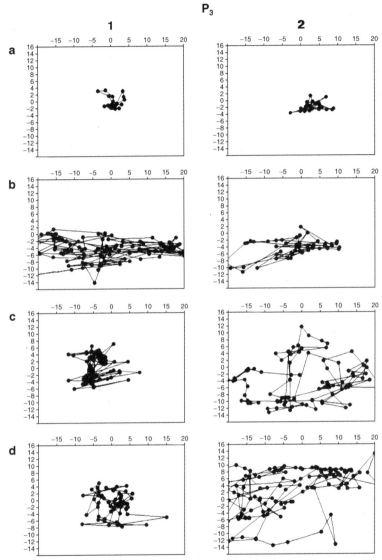

FIG. 5.13 Fixation (a; centre), voluntary saccadic eye movements (b; target distance: 20°), scanning of a dot pattern (Fig. 2.6; c), and scanning of a scene (d; 6 fishermen and a dog, cf. Fig. 6.1), in a patient with Balint's syndrome (P3; see text) before (1) and after (2) practice. Recording time in (a) was 30sec, in (b) 60sec. Scanning times (in seconds): 1: c: 30.6, 2: c: 50.2; 1: d: 33.1, 2: d: 60. 2. Before practice, the patient reported 4 out of 20 dots in (c) and 1 out of 7 items in (d); after practice she reported 9 dots and 4 items, respectively. Note the moderate improvement in fixation accuracy in (2a) and (2b), and the "widening" of the field of oculomotor scanning in (2c) and (2d) which was accompanied, as in case P1 (Fig. 5.10), with an increase in scanning time. For further details, see Figs. 5.1 and 5.3.

TABLE 5.8
Fixation and horizontal saccadic eye movement accuracy in three
patients (P1–P3) with Balint's syndrome before and after practice

	Fixation accuracy (deviation, in °)		Saccadic accuracy (20°)	
	Before M (1SD)	After M (1SD)	Before M (1SD)	After M (1SD)
P1	3.4 (2.2)	1.1 (0.9)	5.5 (3.9)	12.6 (4.2)
P2	3.6 (2.1)	2.6 (1.3)	3.6 (2.2)	15.3 (2.9)
P3	2.1 (3.1)	1.8 (1.1)	5.4 (3.4)	11.4 (3.2)
N	0.5 (0.4)		19.3 (1.4)	

Saccadic localisation of targets was separated by 20°. Fixation was recorded
during 15 sec; 20 saccades were performed to either side. For comparison,
corresponding values of a normal subject (N) of the same age are shown
(cf. Fig. 5.3).

TABLE 5.9
Eye movement parameters in three patients (P1–P3) with Balint's
syndrome before and after practice with visual search tasks

	FIX	FIXr (%)	FD (sec) M (1SD)	A (°) M (1SD)
(A) Dot pattern				
P1				
before	125	60.3	0.51 (0.06)	3.2 (2.2)
after	58	42.4	0.46 (0.12)	4.2 (2.1)
P2				
before	107	64.4	0.32 (0.11)	3.9 (1.6)
after	104	33.6	0.30 (0.06)	5.5 (2.1)
P3				
before	91	65.2	0.24 (0.06)	4.5 (1.3)
after	69	40.7	0.24 (0.07)	5.2 (2.1)
N	26	16.2	0.23 (0.03)	5.6 (2.6)
(B) Scene				
P1				
before	83	67.5	0.44 (0.18)	3.3 (3.2)
after	92	41.3	0.39 (0.11)	5.3 (2.1)
P2				
before	139	62.6	0.32 (0.09)	3.5 (1.4)
after	122	40.2	0.32 (0.06)	4.4 (2.2)
P3				
before	56	51.8	0.26 (0.08)	3.4 (1.1)
after	119	48.7	0.26 (0.09)	5.6 (2.3)
N	54	21.7	0.26 (0.06)	6.4 (2.4)

FIX: number of fixations, FIXr: repetitions of fixations, FD: fixation
duration; A: saccadic amplitudes. For comparison, corresponding values of a
normal subject (N) are shown.

TABLE 5.10
Object and scene identification performance in
three patients (P1–P3) with Balint's syndrome
before and after treatment

	Objects (% correct)		Scenes (% correct)	
	Before	After	Before	After
P1	40.0	87.0	13.3	53.3
P2	20.0	80.0	16.7	70.0
P3	53.3	90.0	26.7	73.3

$n = 30$ trials per category. See text for details.

(cf. Table 5.6). However, even after 940 tachistoscopic presentations we could not find any evidence for an improved reading ability, and we accepted and respected the patient's refusal of further training.

What was the benefit of the intensive training for the patients with Balint's syndrome? Most importantly, all three patients were now able to find their way in familiar surroundings, although all required a relatively long time to find rooms, objects, etc. In less familiar or more complex surroundings such as the far neighbourhood or the supermarket, patients still found visual spatial orientation difficult and feared getting lost. However, one patient (P2) reported that after several trials he was able to more or less get his bearings in this environment. Another patient (P1) preferred the help of his wife. "Why should I make such an effort, when she is willing to help me so nicely?" he convincingly explained to us. The third patient could not regain visual orientation in unfamiliar environments. It remains an open question whether continuing practice would have led to a better outcome in these two patients. Probably patients should be given more practice outside their familiar environments, so that they could better transfer the compensation strategies they have learned to new situations. However, it appears that there is no need to wait for months until patients may eventually recover from Balint's syndrome. Our approach was mainly based on the improvement of visual–spatial abilities which we assumed to be of behavioural relevance in everyday life activities and which represent the basis for more complex activities, e.g. the visual guidance of eye and hand movements, walking, etc. Unfortunately, we did not have a touch screen at the time these patients were treated, but we suppose that systematic practice with visually guided touching would have been a helpful extension of the means of training.

CHAPTER SIX

Visual agnosia

Visual agnosic disorders are impairments in "higher order" or "complex" visual capacities based on both visual–perceptual and visual–cognitive functions and their interactions. Cognition comes into play in nearly every aspect of visual perception, because of the multiple involvement of cognitive capacities such as attention, (working) memory, and planning in the detection, discrimination, identification, and recognition of visual stimuli, and in the visual guidance of motor activities. With respect to diagnostics it is important to differentiate between visual agnosic deficits that are of primary nature and those that are to be explained by deficits in "lower" or elementary visual functions. It was Siemerling (1890) who discussed this issue in detail by demonstrating that a combination of visual field loss, reduced visual acuity, defective colour vision, and disturbed visual scanning can lead to severe impairment of visual identification and recognition. Interestingly, although Siemerling's case report appeared in the same issue of the *Archiv für Psychiatrie und Nervenkrankheiten*, where Lissauer's well-recognised and widely accepted classic case report on visual agnosia was published (Lissauer, 1890), his arguments have not been considered until now (Zihl, 1989). This is even more surprising, since Poppelreuter in 1923 (see Humphreys, Riddoch, & Wallesch, 1996), in a very detailed description, presented a patient exhibiting visual deficits highly similar to those of Lissauer's case and demonstrated convincingly that Lissauer's theory of visual agnosia as a genuine visual recognition disorder cannot be entirely proved by the observations in his own case. According to Lissauer's definition, visual agnosia is a failure to identify or recognise an object visually due to "mistaken identity". Thus, visual agnosia is mainly the misidentification of objects due to similarity of global (e.g. size and shape) or local (e.g. colour, texture, form details) properties, and not a total loss of visual (re-)cognition.

133

Even now there is no unequivocal differentiation between "genuine" visual agnosia and impairments in visual identification and recognition secondary to visual deficits. One has to admit, however, that this differentiation is not an easy task (see Charnallett, Rousset, Carbonnel, & Pellat, 1996; De Haan et al., 1995), since, considering the underlying neural mechanisms (Damasio, Tranel, & Damasio, 1989), a clear distinction between visual perceptual and visual cognitive deficits underlying visual agnosia is rarely possible. It appears reasonable and useful therefore to describe higher-order visual impairments by specifying the various visual and visual–cognitive deficits. Thus, careful and detailed testing and analysis of "lower" and "higher" visual functions is recommended in cases with impaired visual identification and recognition. Such an approach seems all the more appropriate since "pure" visual agnosic disorders are relatively rare. Gloning et al. (1968) found only three cases (< 1%) with visual object agnosia in a group of 241 patients with posterior brain injury, after patients with severe disturbances of "lower" visual functions or mental deterioration were excluded. Furthermore, it is important to point out that language and general intellectual and cognitive functioning have to be preserved at sufficiently high levels so that impairments in these abilities can be excluded as the underlying cause for the failure to identify and recognise objects. In addition, visual agnosia should be restricted to the visual modality, i.e. the patient should be able to correctly recognise an object in another sensory modality. When a patient fails to name visual material but can indicate visual identification and recognition by other means, for example by description or gesture, the failure is considered to result from naming difficulties and not from defective visual identification and recognition.

A clear differentiation between genuine agnosic symptoms and secondary impairments is also of great importance for treatment. It seems evident that in the case of secondarily caused impairments in visual identification and recognition the main approach should be the improvement of the underlying, more elementary visual capacities. As was shown earlier (pp. 16 and 113), visual identification usually returns in these cases without further training after the underlying visual deficits have been reduced due to spontaneous recovery or to specific practice.

FORMS OF VISUAL AGNOSIA

Before presenting observations on the treatment of patients with visual agnosia, it might be useful to describe briefly the main visual cognitive disorders with respect to the visual material that can no longer be correctly recognised by the patient (for a comprehensive description of visual-agnosic disorders, see Benton & Tranel, 1993; Damasio et al., 1989; Grüsser & Landis, 1991; Warrington, 1985). In many cases, category-specific agnosia (i.e. for objects, faces, places, letters) has been reported (see below), but there exist also patients with visual agnosia in more than one visual category (e.g. Ogden, 1993).

Visual object agnosia refers to the difficulty in identifying and recognising objects in the visual modality, while their identification and recognition is preserved in another modality, i.e. when allowed to handle the object or hear its sound when in use. Typically, misidentification results from the incomplete or inappropriate use of object features such as size, shape, or colour. Patients with visual object agnosia very often confuse objects that share the same or familiar features and do not consider that the feature(s) they are using may not be (sufficiently) characteristic of the object in question. In addition, patients may be unaware that they are disregarding other object features that may help to correctly identify and recognise an individual object. Thus, the main visual–cognitive deficit in visual object agnosia is apparently the impairment in the selection and integration of features that characterise an individual object and enable its differentiation from similar objects. Furthermore, supervisory processes that are used to control the result of identification and recognition and that allow a procedure to be registered as faulty, appear to be absent or at least reduced (Damasio et al., 1989; Zihl & von Cramon, 1986b).

Patients with *prosopagnosia* have lost the ability to visually recognise familiar faces and to learn new faces (Damasio et al., 1989). Although it is often stated that prosopagnosia is a selective visual disorder, the majority of prosopagnosic patients reported in the literature also exhibited difficulties with the visual recognition of other familiar objects, e.g. animals, buildings, or cars. However, difficulties with the visual recognition of familiar faces are typically more prominent. It appears, of course, more striking when patients can no longer recognise the face of their spouse, their children, or even their own face in a mirror or on a photograph than when visual recognition of an object is impaired to the same degree. Usually prosopagnosic patients can correctly identify familiar people by their voice, their body movements, or their dress. If a patient shows a more moderate form of this visual disorder, the differentiation of faces that look very similar, i.e. share common features, may be difficult and such faces may therefore be easily confused.

The term *topographical agnosia* is often used to describe various difficulties with geographical orientation either in the real world or on maps, or both. Patients have problems with orientation in their familiar environments and can neither make use of maps, nor draw a plan of a well-known route, their house, or their living room. Sometimes patients complain of getting lost even in familiar places or environments because these places and environments are "stripped" of their familiarity (environmental agnosia). Difficulties with geographical orientation and environmental agnosia often occur in association, but can also occur individually.

Patients with *(pure) alexia* have problems identifying individual letters and/ or building words out of letters ("letter-by-letter-reading"). The term "pure" refers to the fact that reading difficulties in these cases are not part of an aphasic syndrome. The severity of alexia may depend on the print typeface of letters and words. Reading of hand-written words, even of the patient's own, is usually more impaired than the identification of letters or the reading of words in distinct print. In contrast to patients suffering from dyslexia due to parafoveal field loss or to visual neglect, patients with alexia do not benefit from vertical word presentation.

SPONTANEOUS RECOVERY

Only few reports exist of spontaneous recoveries from visual agnosia. Adler (1944, 1950) reported minimal recovery in 5 years in a patient with severe visual agnosic symptoms due to carbon monoxide poisoning. About 40 years later, this patient was retested in detail by Sparr, Jay, Drislane, and Venna (1991). Visual agnosic deficits still existed, including visual object agnosia, prosopagnosia, alexia, and impaired visual imagery. In addition, visual–spatial disorientation was also persistent. Sparr et al. pointed out that carbon monoxide poisoning induces complex visual deficits with a very poor prognosis. Kertesz (1979) presented follow-up data on a patient with visual agnosia, who had suffered traumatic brain injury in a car accident. Visual agnosia persisted for more than 10 years without significant recovery. Wilson and Davidoff (1993) retested a patient with visual agnosia 10 years after she had sustained severe head injury in an accident. These authors found recovery from visual agnosia for real objects and some improvement for the identification of other classes of visual stimuli (photographs of objects and faces, drawings of objects, letters). In a patient suffering from prosopagnosia, Bruyer et al. (1983) observed no recovery over a 12-month period of observation.

TREATMENT

Poppelreuter (1917/1990) was the first to treat patients with visual agnosic symptoms. His method of training was mainly based on teaching patients the features which are characteristic or even unique for a particular object and to use and rely on these features. Poppelreuter found some improvement in three out of six cases with visual agnosia.

Of course, patients exhibiting difficulties with visual recognition may be told to use context information and non-visual cues about objects, faces, buildings, or locations, or may do so spontaneously. Nevertheless, it might be of interest to know whether the severity of visual agnosia can be reduced by specific practice, and which procedure(s) may be helpful in achieving this goal.

In an attempt to improve the functions and processes underlying visual identification and recognition, we developed training techniques similar to those used by Poppelreuter (1917/1990). As in the case with training of colour discrimination (see p. 102) and based on experiments showing that errorless learning is superior to errorful learning (Sidman & Stoddard, 1967; Wilson, Baddeley, Evans, & Shiel, 1994; Wilson & Evans, 1996) we adopted a treatment strategy preventing guessing and permitting only correct responses. In the two patients who are reported here, visual agnosia occurred after bilateral occipitotemporal infarction in one case (P1) and after closed head trauma accompanied by severe chronic hypoxia in the other (P2; same patient as P2 on p. 102). Both patients showed left-sided hemianopia with field sparing of 3° in P1, and 2° in P2. Visual acuity was 1.0 in both cases. Neither patient complained of "blurred" vision; spatial contrast sensitivity was in the normal range. P2 also exhibited cerebral dyschromatopsia. Visual agnosia persisted in P1 for 15 weeks and in P2 for 22 months without significant recovery. In both patients, visual recognition of all types of visual material, i.e. objects, faces, and letters was affected, although to varying degrees (Table 6.1). With respect to faces, not only recognition of familiar faces was severely affected, but also identification of gender and age. Identification of facial expression was preserved. Patients did not show other cognitive impairments, except for a moderate memory problem for verbal material in P2. Figure 6.1 shows eye movement recordings during scanning of a dot pattern, of a scene, and of faces in a normal control subject. In Fig. 6.2 eye movement recordings of the two patients with visual agnosia are shown. Patients' oculomotor scanning of the dot pattern was characterised by visual disorientation and elevated scanning times. Oculomotor scanning of faces was even more impaired, and patients were unable to report the faces correctly. P1 identified the face of a young man (Fig. 6.2, d) as a "young girl with dark skin", P2 as "a middle-aged woman". Both patients had great difficulties identifying the two faces (Fig. 6.2, e) as belonging to the same person.

In our attempt to improve patients' prerequisites to identify visual material, we first trained oculomotor scanning (for methods, see pp. 48 and 61) because both patients suffered from homonymous visual field loss and visual disorientation.

TABLE 6.1

Visual object and scene identification and recognition performance (number of correctly identified items) in two patients (P1, P2) with homonymous hemianopia and visual agnosia before and after practice with visual scanning and visual orientation. See text for further details

Object categories	No. of items in category	P1		P2	
		Before	After	Before	After
Food	30	3	4	5	4
Personal hygiene articles	20	2	4	1	3
Clothing and shoes	30	1	3	2	2
Animals	30	1	3	2	4
Famous faces	20	0	0	0	0
Familiar faces	10	0	3	0	0
Letters	20	3	3	0	0
Scenes	30	0	2	0	1

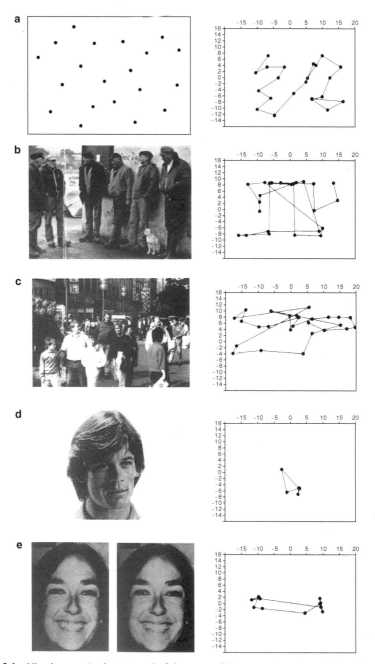

FIG. 6.1 Visual scenes (a: dot pattern; b: fishermen and dog; c: market place; d: face of a young male; e: two identical faces of a middle-aged female) and oculomotor scanning patterns in a normal control subject who reported correctly 20 dots (a) and identified correctly the scenes and faces. Scanning times (in seconds): a: 8.5, b: 11.7, c: 10.9, d: 2.6, e: 4.6. x-axis: horizontal extension of stimulus array (in degress; 0 = centre, negative values left, positive values right), y-axis: vertical extension (0 = centre, negative values down, positive values up). Dots indicate fixation locations.

138

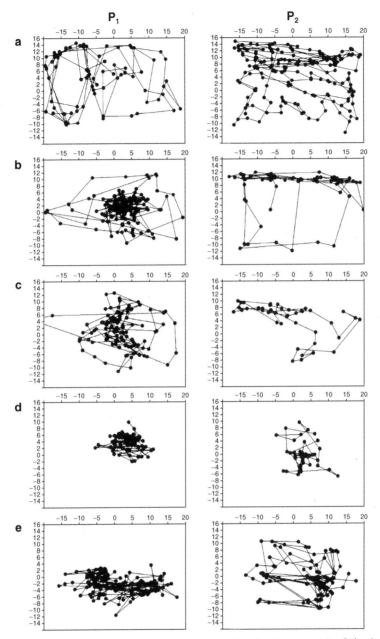

FIG. 6.2 Oculomotor scanning patterns during the scanning of a dot pattern (a), of visual scenes (b and c), of one (d) and of two identical (e) human faces in two patients (P1, P2) with visual agnosia. Scanning times (in seconds): P1: a: 32.4, b: 60.3, c: 42.4, d: 30.8, e: 91.3; P2: a: 58.1, b: 40.2, c: 25.9, d: 19.1, e: 44.1. Scenes as in Fig. 6.1. Both patients eventually reported correctly the dots (a) and the items in the two scenes (b, c), but could not identify the face in (d) (P1: "possibly male"; P2: "young lady"), and the faces in (e) (P1: "probably twin sisters"; P2: "different women"). For further details, see Fig. 6.1.

139

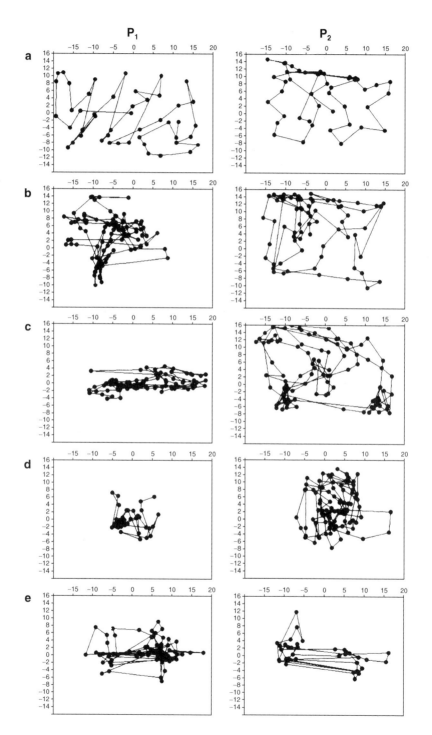

Both patients gained an effective oculomotor compensation (see Fig. 6.3), which, however, did not improve visual identification and recognition (Table 6.1). Patient 2 was then given intensive practice with colours (see p. 102), since he often used colours to identify objects, but had great difficulties with colour hues. Typical confusions were, for example, apple and orange, or cheese and butter; in both cases, shape and size are too similar to allow accurate identification. After improved colour discrimination was achieved (see Fig. 4.4 p. 105), we started with practice of the selection and use of object features to enhance visual identification and recognition in both cases. A detailed analysis of the errors in visual identification and recognition (Table 6.2) revealed that both patients either disregarded features, and used only one feature, or selected a feature that was not really characteristic of the object in question. For example, when shown greenish fruits with a round shape, P2 always "identified" them as "apples", which in one sense is correct, but there are also green tomatoes (before becoming ripe), green pears, green peppers, etc. Or he called all yellow fluids "beer", not considering that fruit juices, for example orange or pineapple juice, are also this colour. Similar errors were observed with faces; the patient mainly used hair length as the essential feature for differentiating males and females. However, since males may have long hair and females may have their hair cut short, this feature is no longer unequivocally valid for differentiating gender. Of course, faulty selection and omission of features are in principle not to be considered independent error types. A subject may choose only one object feature and not necessarily the (most) characteristic one. Other features should therefore be considered too but if they are not then visual identification will often be faulty. What is missing are the cognitive processes to "supervise" selection of features and to control the result of identification, based on plausibility and derived from experience. In the third phase of practice we therefore concentrated on teaching the patients to select visual object features, to check the selected feature(s) with respect to the value for correct identification, and finally to examine the outcome of identification in terms of correct, partly correct, and false responses, with immediate feedback. If, for example, a coloured photograph of a red tomato is shown, the response "red tomato" would be the correct answer, "a red round fruit" would be a partly correct answer, "an apple" or "a small red ball" would be incorrect responses.

FIG. 6.3 (opposite) Oculomotor scanning patterns after practice with visual search in two patients (P1 and P2 in Fig. 6.2) with visual agnosia during the scanning of a dot pattern (a), of visual scenes (b, c), of one (d) and of two (e) human faces. Same scenes as in Fig. 6.1. Dot counting was now correct in both patients as was the report of items for scenes (b) and (c). In contrast, neither patient could identify with certainty the face in (d) or the two faces in (e) as identical. Scanning times (in seconds): P1: a: 27.2, b: 56.1, c: 39.7, d: 36.3, e: 31.4; P2: a: 16.1, b: 32.2, c: 42.7, d: 36.1, e: 25.9. Note the reduction in scanning times for the dot patterns while scanning times for scenes and faces remained more or less the same. For further details, see Fig. 6.1.

TABLE 6.2
Types and frequencies of visual recognition errors in two patients
(P1, P2) with visual agnosia (cf. Table 6.1)

	Response	
Item	*P1*	*P2*
"Global" features		
Apple		A reddish ball
Letters		Vertically put plates
Mirror (rectangular)	Whitish modern house	
Camera	Television screen	Washing machine
Raspberries	Red apples	
Black chocolate		Connected dark bricks
Potatoes		Huge dirty stones
Slices of bread	Sandals	
Dog	Cow	Big animal
Banana	Yellowish tree	A yellow reed
"Local" feature		
Knife (with wooden grip)	A piece of wood	A metal mirror
Watch	Two black lines	Something written
Potatoes	Pieces of earth	
Rice		Small white buttons
Bicycle	Two balls	
Ties	Coloured patterns	
Swiss cheese		Holes in a wall
Horse	Lion	
Frequency of error types		
(n = 100 items)		
"Global" errors	36%	26%
"Local" errors	48%	62%
"Mixed" errors	16%	12%

Table 6.3 contains the plan for treatment and the number of trials in each phase. To assess practice and generalisation effects, we used the objects mentioned previously in Table 6.1 before and after practice. Typically, between two and four sessions, 45 minutes each, were carried out each day. Photographs of visual objects and faces were shown for an unlimited time in blocks of 15–20 stimuli each. Patients were instructed to first inspect the whole object and to report all features they could find. Then they were to select the feature(s) they believed to be the most characteristic one(s) of the particular object, to check the result, and then to identify the object. Patients were forced always to follow this procedure in order to develop a systematic strategy for visual identification and also to prevent hasty responses. Table 6.4 shows the results after practice. In addition to the improvement in the trained object class, there was some generalisation to other classes of visual objects, except for letters and familiar faces. The

TABLE 6.3
Plan of treatment in two patients (P1, P2) with visual
agnosia (errorless identification and recognition learning)

	No. of trials	
	P1	P2
Object categories		
Food (50 items)		
Clothing and shoes (50 items)		
Animals (40 items)		
Practice procedures		
Information processing:		
Complete report of object attributes	1630	2040
Information selection:		
Selection of features which are		
characteristic for a particular object	1440	3024
"Hypothesis testing":		
Development and use of cognitive strategies		
to supervise and control visual identification	1620	3860

TABLE 6.4
Improvement of visual identification (number of correct responses) in two patients
(P1, P2) with visual agnosia after practice with visual information processing,
selection, and cognitive control (see Table 6.3)

		P1		P2	
Object categories	*No. of items in category*	*Before*	*After*	*Before*	*After*
Food	30	4	22	4	19
Personal hygiene articles	20	4	14	1	9
Clothing and shoes	30	3	18	2	21
Animals	30	3	18	2	14
Famous faces	20	0	2	0	0
Familiar faces	10	3	5	0	1
Letters	20	3	5	0	2
Scenes	30	0	17	0	13

improvement in the identification process was also associated, at least in part, with an improvement in oculomotor scanning of objects and faces (Fig. 6.4).

Since the identification of letters and familiar faces was not found to have improved, we continued with specific practice concerning these stimulus classes. We started with pairs of capital letters that look quite different (I and O; A and D) and continued with letters that look more similar, but are still clearly distinct

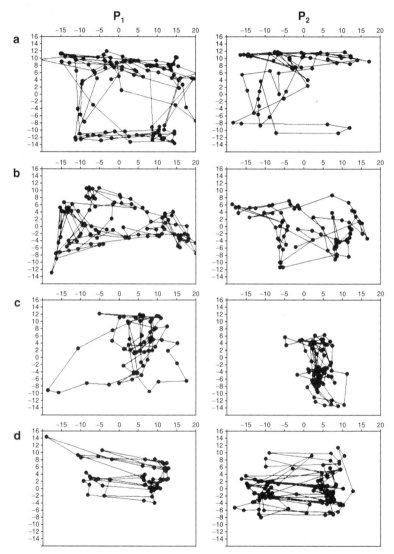

FIG. 6.4 Oculomotor scanning patterns after practice with selection and identification of visual stimulus features in two patients (P1 and P2 in Fig. 6.2) with visual agnosia during the scanning of visual scenes (a, b), of one (c) and of two (d) human faces. Same scenes as in Fig. 6.1. Both patients reported correctly the items for the two scenes (a, b), and could now also correctly identify the faces in (c) and (d). Scanning times (in seconds): P1: a: 45.7, b: 45.4, c: 30.3, d: 22.9; P2: a: 27.5; b: 42.1; c: 31.0; d: 51.1. Note that in both patients the improvement in visual identification was accompanied by an increase in scanning time (cf. Fig. 6.3). For further details, see Fig. 6.1.

(I and H; B and D). Finally, we used letter pairs that differed with respect to one feature only (I and T; O and C). After intensive practice with all letters and with numbers from 1–10 (about 40–60 trials for each character), we found considerable improvement in the identification of all characters, but accuracy of recognition differed between items (see Table 6.5). Interestingly, and also surprisingly, patients could correctly read whole words after the improvement in character identification, although slowly and somewhat with hesitation, indicating that they did not suffer from alexia, at least not in a severe form, because integration of individual letters into words was possible without further practice.

A similar procedure was used to improve patients' capacity to differentiate and use facial features. Both patients benefited from this practice, both in terms of correct responses (Table 6.6) and of oculomotor scanning (Fig. 6.4 and Table 6.7). At this time P1 was discharged from hospital; practice with reading was continued by a speech therapist at home. With P2 we continued practice of reading using tachistoscopic presentation of words on a monitor (see p. 81). After an additional 30 sessions P2 could read more fluently, but his reading performance (55 wpm) was still considerably below the range of age-matched normal control subjects (148–186 wpm). His reading eye movements were also found to have improved, and were now more regular than before practice (Fig. 6.5).

Finally, we tried to improve visual recognition of familiar faces and learning of new faces in P2. We did this by first giving the patient practice in differentiating faces on the basis of correct selection of facial features and using the same procedure as with the identification of objects. This practice led to an improvement in visual face discrimination but not in visual recognition of familiar faces

TABLE 6.5
Practice with the identification of letters in two patients (P1, P2) with visual agnosia: Procedure of treatment and outcome

			Results (% correct)			
	No. of trials		P1		P2	
	P1	P2	Before	After	Before	After
Procedure of practice						
Discrimination and identification of:						
Letters with very low similarity (e.g. I–O)	980	1660				
Letters sharing similar features (e.g. I–T)	1160	2140				
Letters with high similarity (e.g. E–F)	740	1540				
Results						
Letter categories (50 items per category)						
Low similarity			8	6	4	82
Medium similarity			2	52	0	72
High similarity			0	32	0	56

TABLE 6.6
Practice with the discrimination and identification of unfamiliar faces in two
patients (P1, P2) with visual agnosia: Procedure of treatment and outcome

| | No. of trials | | Results (% correct) | | | |
| | | | P1 | | P2 | |
	P1	P2	Before	After	Before	After
Procedure of practice						
Discrimination and identification of:						
Age (child, youngster, middle-aged, old)	260	580				
Gender (female, male)	160	440				
Facial expression (sad, happy, neutral)	120	180				
Results						
Categories (30 per category)						
Age			53	87	20	73
Gender			60	97	37	80
Facial expression			63	97	70	93
Familiar faces ($n = 10$)			5	9	1	2

(see Table 6.6). For example, he could now quite often correctly identify his father's face by vision alone; this was because meanwhile he had learned to use his father's bald head as a characteristic feature for identification. If he was shown the face only, he was still unable to recognise him. We used a technique for associating familiar faces and their corresponding names in both directions (face → name; name → face). Ten photographs of the faces of family members and of close friends were used along with their names. The outcome after 100 trials (10 per face) was not very promising (Table 6.8), although there was some improvement. It may be important to note that during the period of practice with faces (three consecutive weeks) the patient could not be persuaded to use vision exclusively or at least predominantly for the recognition of familiar faces. He still relied on voices and the use of context, which enabled him immediately and correctly to recognise family members and friends. The successful substitution of the severely impaired visual recognition of familiar faces and the learning of new faces through the acoustic modality and by (visual) context information, which now could be more effectively used, is a good example that the balance between the costs (a long lasting, highly demanding training) and the outcome (a "significant", but behaviourally often irrelevant improvement) is an important issue to be considered in the planning and procurement of rehabilitation measures. Patients with visual agnosia may regain the ability to perform quite complex activities without recovery of visual–cognitive functions, but by using context information and non-visual cues in a highly effective way.

TABLE 6.7
Eye movement parameters in two patients (P1, P2) with visual agnosia
before treatment (A), after practice with oculomotor scanning (B), and
after practice with selection and integration of object features (C)

	FIX	FIXr (%)	FD (sec)	A (°)
P1 (A)				
Dot pattern	79	36.7	0.20	4.5
Scene 1	139	62.2	0.32	3.7
Scene 2	103	49.5	0.30	4.1
Face 1	67	70.1	0.26	4.1
Face 2	149	69.8	0.30	3.2
P1 (B)				
Dot pattern	47	14.9	0.26	6.6
Scene 1	95	55.8	0.40	3.9
Scene 2	92	66.3	0.31	3.1
Face 1	43	60.5	0.40	3.5
Face 2	81	58.0	0.30	3.7
P1 (C)				
Scene 1	69	30.9	0.26	5.5
Scene 2	73	34.7	0.28	4.9
Face 1	64	40.6	0.30	4.9
Face 2	52	46.2	0.26	4.7
P2 (A)				
Dot pattern	165	46.1	0.26	3.8
Scene 1	66	46.1	0.33	5.9
Scene 2	42	35.7	0.32	4.1
Face 1	45	46.7	0.22	4.1
Face 2	97	54.6	0.24	4.7
P2 (B)				
Dot pattern	45	20.0	0.36	5.0
Scene 1	73	44.2	0.30	4.2
Scene 2	108	44.4	0.30	3.9
Face 1	55	53.7	0.28	4.1
Face 2	88	52.6	0.25	4.2
P2 (C)				
Scene 1	51	31.4	0.24	6.5
Scene 2	73	33.8	0.28	4.8
Face 1	79	36.4	0.28	3.5
Face 2	69	33.5	0.26	4.8
N				
Dot pattern	22	13.6	0.24	5.6
Scene 1	23	21.7	0.26	6.9
Scene 2	29	31.0	0.26	7.3
Face 1	6	0	0.22	4.6
Face 2	10	0	0.28	6.3

FIX: number of fixations, FIXr: repetition of fixations, FD: mean fixation
durations, A: mean saccadic amplitudes. For comparison, corresponding values of a
male normal subject (N) aged 52 years are shown. Tasks (see Fig. 6.1): scanning of
a dot pattern, of two scenes (1,2), of a single face (face 1), and comparison of two
identical faces (face 2). See text for details.

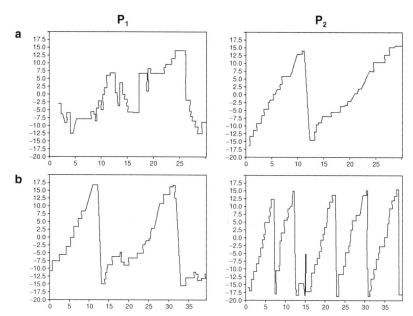

FIG. 6.5 Reading eye movements in two patients with visual agnosia (P1, P2; same as in Figs. 6.2–6.4) before (a) and after (b) practice. Reading performance: P1: a: 7 wpm, b: 18 wpm; P2: a: 24 wpm; b: 47 wpm. Note the reappearance of regular reading eye movements after practice, especially in P2. x-axis: time period of recording (in seconds), y-axis: horizontal extension of line (in degrees). 0 = centre, negative values left, positive values right.

TABLE 6.8
Practice with the identification and naming of familiar faces in a patient (P2) with visual agnosia: Procedure of treatment and outcome ($n = 55$ for discrimination, and 30 for identification in each category)

		Results (% correct)	
	No. of trials	Before	After
*Procedure of practice**			
Discrimination between pairs of faces	600		
Identification of faces (including naming)	140 (per face)		
Discrimination		66	96
Identification			
Own face		13	17
Mother		13	23
Father		20	53
Aunt		7	27
Uncle		13	30

*Stimuli: patient's own face; faces of mother and father; faces of closest aunt and uncle.

148

We instructed our patients to further use their regained visual identification capacities after remission. When tested 6 months later, we found evidence for further improvement in the identification of objects, faces, scenes, and in reading (Table 6.9). P2 however still suffers from severe prosopagnosia.

In conclusion, patients with visual agnosia can be treated successfully, although the data presented here have the character of preliminary observations. As with other complex visual disorders, it seems a useful procedure first to assess the impaired as well as the preserved visual functions and abilities and then to develop a plan of treatment starting with the improvement of "low-level" visual capacities. A further help is generalisation of treatment effects, for example, the transfer of effective selection of features from one class of visual objects to others. If successful, generalisation can considerably reduce the amount of practice. However, whether or not generalisation takes place has to be tested in each individual case. Although there is evidence that visual cognition is organised in a modular form (Gainotti, Silveri, Daniele, & Giustolisi, 1995; McCarthy & Warrington, 1988; Powell & Davidoff, 1995; Small, Hart, Nguyen, & Gordon, 1995), we still do not know very much about the association and dissociation of visual cognitive capacities. A good example is the case of a visually agnosic artist reported by Wapner, Judd, and Gardner (1978). This patient regained his ability to make drawings characteristic of his premorbid artwork despite a persisting severe deficit in visual recognition. The search for further evidence on the basis of recovery of visual–cognitive capacities can therefore also provide important insight into the brain organisation of more complex visual functions, including visual knowledge.

Finally, especially with respect to complex visual functions, we have to differentiate between an improvement as assessed by a measure of performance and the "ecological" value of this improvement, i.e. its significance in terms of reduction of the degree of visual disability in everyday life. In our two patients, visual object discrimination (based on feature selection) and object recognition could be improved such that the degree of the visual disability was clearly

TABLE 6.9
Follow-up (6 months post-treatment) in two patients (P1, P2) with visual agnosia

	Objects (% correct)	FamF	Scenes (% correct)	Reading (wpm)
P1				
End of treatment	65.5	9	56.7	11
Follow-up	86.0	10	90.0	69
P2				
End of treatment	57.3	2	43.3	55
Follow-up	70.9	3	53.3	113

Visual object identification (10 out of 4 categories, cf. Table 6.4; $n = 40$), recognition of familiar faces (FamF; $n = 10$), identification of scenes ($n = 30$), and reading (wpm: words per minute).

reduced, i.e. there was a considerable "ecological" value in this improvement. In contrast, P2 did not benefit from practising familiar face recognition, although visual face discrimination could be improved. Thus, the increase in test scores on visual face recognition was of only low "ecological" value if at all.

CHAPTER SEVEN

Central scotoma

Patients with central scotoma suffer from a variety of visual impairments, depending on the size of the central scotoma and the associated visual disorders. The reduction or loss of the central portion of the visual field is typically associated with a more or less severe impairment of visual spatial contrast sensitivity, visual acuity, reading, and form, object, and face perception. The relative or total loss of foveal vision also means that patients have lost the central landmark of the visual field that serves as a reference point for optimal fixation and the straight-ahead direction. As a consequence, they are unable to accurately fixate a visual stimulus, to shift their gaze accurately from one object to another, to scan a scene or a face appropriately, or to guide their eye movements during reading properly. Furthermore, they are unable to see a stimulus as a whole; when shifting their fixation to better perceive an object, they may lose it. "When looking directly at objects or people I cannot see them, because they are no longer there, and I cannot find anything, even when I shift my gaze", as one patient described it. They find it extremely difficult to get their bearings in rooms or places, and report getting "completely lost" when scanning a word or a scene. In our experience, patients with central scotoma are aware of their pronounced visual handicaps.

There exists no systematic experience concerning the recovery from central scotoma, nor is there a kind of systematic treatment known which could reduce the various visual impairments in these patients. It appears that spontaneous recovery is rather limited in patients with central scotoma due to postchiasmatic injury (Teuber et al., 1960; Walsh & Hoyt, 1969). An exception to these findings are patients suffering from central scotoma associated with multiple sclerosis. These patients may eventually in part or even fully recover from central scotoma;

however, the loss of vision in these cases is typically of prechiasmatic origin (e.g. Slamovits, Rosen, Cheng, & Striph, 1991).

The main question concerning a possibly effective procedure of treatment is whether the various deficits in visual form and object perception represent genuine disorders, or whether they are secondarily caused by the loss or at least severe reduction of foveal visual capacities, including visual localisation and visual guidance of eye (and hand) movements.

Figure 7.1 shows the visual field plots of six patients; in Table 7.1 the various visual disorders found in these patients are summarised. Binocular visual form acuity was 0.05 in three patients, and 0.20 in one case. In two patients, no type of acuity could be measured. Form and object perception and reading were

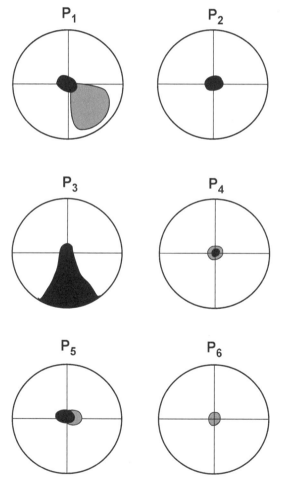

FIG. 7.1   Binocular visual field plots in 6 patients (P1–P6 in Table 7.1) with central scotoma. Black areas indicate absolute, grey areas amblyopic defects.

TABLE 7.1

Clinical details and visual deficits in six patients with central scotoma.
All patients suffered their deficits after chronic cerebral hypoxia

Clinical details and visual deficits	P1	P2	P3	P4	P5	P6
Age (years)	26	28	48	21	36	19
Gender	F	M	F	M	F	F
Time post-injury (weeks)	16	9	11	28	52	8
Acuity	0.05	?	0.05	0.05	?	0.22
"Blurred vision"	+	—	+	—	—	+
Colour vision	(–)	(–)	+	(–)	(–)	(–)
Object vision	—	—	(+)	(+)	—	(+)
Visual-spatial orientation	—	—	(–)	—	—	(+)
Neglect	–	–	–	–	–	–
Attention	(–)	(–)	+	+	+	+
Memory	(–)	(–)	+	(–)	+	+
Language	(–)	+	+	+	+	+
Anosognosia	–	+	–	–	–	–

+: preserved, (+): partly preserved (e.g. crude form vision), – impaired, (–) partly impaired, —: absent or lost. Acuity is given in binocular Snellen fractions. ?: no data available.

TABLE 7.2

Visual identification in six patients with central scotoma (for visual fields, see Fig. 7.1). Forms, faces and letters were shown in black and white, the other objects were on coloured photographs

Category	P1 (% correct)	P2 (% correct)	P3 (% correct)	P4 (% correct)	P5 (% correct)	P6 (% correct)
Forms (n = 30)	6.7	3.3	6.7	3.3	0.0	26.7
Fruit (n = 30)	13.3	6.7	6.7	10.0	3.3	53.3
Tools (n = 30)	6.7	3.3	3.3	6.7	0.0	30.0
Faces (n = 30)	0.0	6.7	0.0	3.3	0.0	16.7
Letters (n = 30)	3.3	3.3	0.0	3.3	6.7	36.7

Stimuli used: Geometrical forms: circle, triangle, star, rectangle, bar, cross (size: 3cm); Fruit: apple, bear, banana, grapes, cherries, orange (size of total figure: 6–8cm); Tools: hammer, spoon, comb, knife, pencil, scissors (size of total figure: 6–8cm); Faces: boy, girl; middle-aged woman and man, old woman and man (size of total figure: 6–8cm); Letters: A, C, D, E, S (size: 2cm).

limited to "crude" impressions even when large simple shapes, objects or letters were used. As a consequence, visual identification was more or less at the level of guessing (Table 7.2). When looking at objects or faces, all patients exhibited a similarly strange behaviour: They shifted their head to the left or right to bring the object in question as close as possible to the border of the scotoma where form vision was best. This strategy is underlined by the recordings of saccadic eye movements (see Fig. 7.2). Patients fixated the visual stimulus directly but failed to find the actual stimulus location by several degrees.

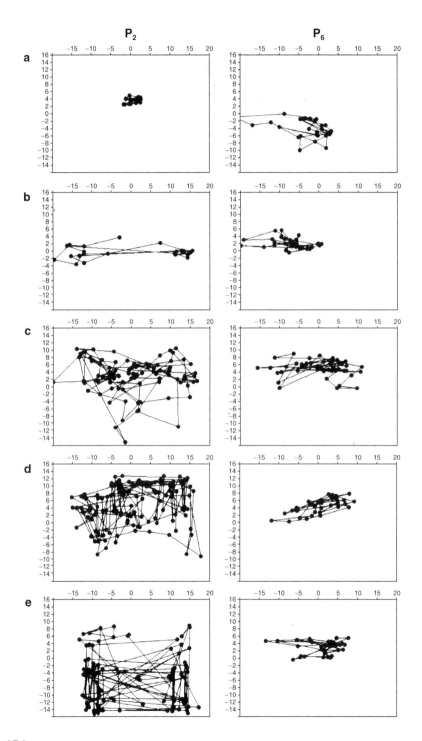

TABLE 7.3
Plan of treatment of visual disorders in patients with central scotoma

Phase	Treatment
1	*Fixation and saccadic localisation* Fixating real objects and touching them; locating targets in the perimeter
2	*Oculomotor scanning (overview, visual orientation)* Visual search tasks using large objects (diameter = 2.5–4.3°)
3	*Contrast sensitivity and form discrimination* Detection of spatial contrasts; discrimination of simple forms
4	*Reading (only in two patients)* Reading words presented tachistoscopically; practice with reading of text material

For the treatment of these patients a special plan of practice was developed which comprised the visual guidance of eye movements, visual–spatial orientation, and foveal capacities including contrast sensitivity, form discrimination, and reading (Table 7.3). In a first attempt to remediate these patients' visual disabilities we attempted to improve saccadic localisation. The procedure of practice in saccadic localisation was similar to that used in patients with visual field defects (see p. 37) and in the patient with severe impairment in visual space perception after bilateral posterior parietal injury (see p. 110), with the main intention to improve fixation accuracy. For this reason, presentation time was unlimited, i.e. the target disappeared only when the patient indicated fixating it. Figure 7.3 shows the result of saccadic localisation before and after practice in two patients (P2 and P4 in Table 7.1 and Fig. 7.1). While P2 could fixate the target quite accurately after about 900 trials, P2 required about twice the number of trials (1720), before his localisation accuracy improved. Table 7.4 shows the improvement in saccadic localisation accuracy after treatment. However, most of the patients still exhibited a systematic localisation error which ranged from 1.5–4°, with undershoots being more frequent than overshoots. Perimetric testing after this practice did not reveal any obvious changes in the extent of the scotoma in either patient.

FIG. 7.2 (opposite) Fixation (a; centre), voluntary saccadic eye movements (b), scanning of a dot pattern (c; see Fig. 6.1a), scanning of a scene (d; see Fig. 6.1b), and of two human faces (see Fig. 6.1e) in two patients with central scotomata (P2 and P6 in Fig. 7.1). Recording times in (a) and (b) were 30sec. Mean fixation deviation was 3° for P6, and 7° for P3. Scanning times (in seconds): P2: c: 63.0, d: 76.4, e: 66.2; P6: c: 34.5, d: 31.3, e: 31.8. P2 reported 11 out of 20 dots (c), P6 16 dots. In (d) P2 reported 2 out of 7 items, P6 4 items. P6 could eventually identify the two faces in (e) as identical, while P2 could not. a, c–e: x-axis: horizontal extension of stimulus array (in degress; 0 = centre, negative values left, positive values right), y-axis: vertical extension (0 = centre, negative values down, positive values up). Dots indicate fixation locations. b: Bottom left, top right. x-axis: time period of recording (in seconds); y-axis: horizontal amplitude (in degrees) of saccades (0 = centre).

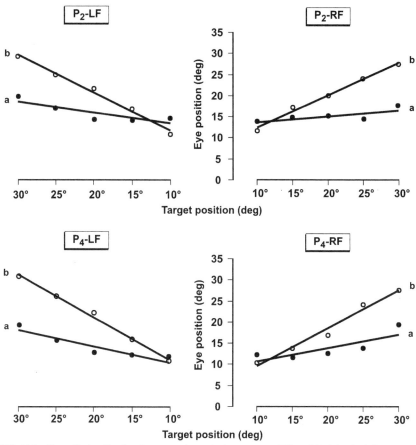

FIG. 7.3   Saccadic localisation (means and standard errors; n = 10/condition) in the left (LF) and right (RF) hemifields in two patients with central scotoma (P2 and P4 in Table 7.1 and in Fig. 7.2) before (a) and after (b) practice. Bottom: left, top: right. x-axis: time period of recording (seconds); y-axis: horizontal amplitude (in degrees) of saccades (0 = centre). Note the improved correspondence between target and eye positions after practice.

Despite the improvement in saccadic localisation and the concomitant improvement in finding objects in space all patients still reported difficulties with the overview and with visual orientation. Treatment was therefore continued with systematic scanning of stimulus arrays on slides similar to those used with other patient groups suffering from homonymous visual field loss (see p. 48). However, arrays contained fewer (3–15) and larger stimuli (2.7° in diameter). Because of the still impaired visual acuity, we used only squares, crosses and circles as stimuli. Patients were asked to obtain, first of all, a global view, and to find out the position of the stimuli and to indicate them using a light pointer before identifying them. In a first step, they were asked to find one (e.g. a cross)

TABLE 7.4

Outcome of practice with saccadic localisation in the Tübingen perimeter in six patients with central scotoma: Mean distances ($n = 10$ per position) from target positions (10°, 20°, and 30°) in the left and right hemifields

| | Left hemifield | | Right hemifield | | |
	Before M (1SD)	After M (1SD)	Before M (1SD)	After M (1SD)	No. of trials
P1	−5.0 (2.2)	−0.9 (0.7)	−4.3 (2.7)	−1.3 (0.9)	1300
P2	−8.5 (4.8)	−3.8 (2.6)	−6.7 (5.9)	−4.1 (2.7)	1600
P3	−6.1 (3.6)	−1.5 (0.4)	+7.1 (3.9)	−2.3 (1.4)	1350
P4	−6.6 (3.2)	−0.4 (1.9)	−5.9 (3.6)	+0.5 (2.1)	1400
P5	−4.3 (3.0)	+2.2 (1.1)	−5.1 (2.6)	+3.1 (1.6)	1300
P6	+2.4 (0.8)	−0.8 (0.3)	−3.1 (1.3)	+0.9 (0.4)	600
N	−1.1 (0.8)		−0.8 (0.6)		

+: overshoot, −: undershoot. Corresponding data of 10 age-matched normal control subjects (N) are shown for comparison.

target among nontargets (e.g. circles). The number of nontargets was stepwise increased from 3 to 10; the number of targets from 1 to 5. Searching time was used as a response measure. After practice patients showed a considerable reduction in the time required in both the search and the dot scanning tests (Table 7.5). The fact that this reduction in time was mainly due to an improvement in the overview and in visual orientation becomes evident from the eye movement recordings in two patients (see Figs. 7.4 and 7.5). Both patients showed a more systematic oculomotor scanning pattern after practice, with less fixations and refixations, and a better spatial organisation of their scanpath.

Visual acuity, form discrimination, and visual recognition of objects and letters were tested before and after practice of fixation and oculomotor scanning. We hypothesised that if visual discrimination and recognition is primarily impaired in these patients because of their inaccurate fixation and scanning, then they should perform better after practice. As Table 7.6 shows, visual acuity, form vision, and object, face, and letter recognition were indeed all improved after practice although the degree of improvement varied considerably between patients and stimulus categories.

Three patients (P1, P3, and P6 in Table 7.1 and Fig. 7.1) reported "blurred" vision, which is typically associated with impaired contrast vision (see p. 92). We measured spatial contrast sensitivity in these patients. In two patients contrast sensitivity was considerably reduced, in one case it was moderately impaired (Fig. 7.6). We decided therefore to give the three patients specific practice (for method of measurement and procedure of practice, see p. 94). We found an improvement in two patients (P1, P6; Fig. 7.6), which was accompanied with an increase in visual acuity (Snellen fractions before practice: P1 = 0.29,

TABLE 7.5

Practice with visual search (using slides and the search-paradigm) in six patients with central scotoma: search performance in a visual search and a scanning task

	No. of trials	Before	After
Search task			
Time (sec)			
P1	1620	128.4	45.7
P2	1980	216.1	88.4
P3	1380	88.9	43.5
P4	1460	108.3	27.8
P5	960	186.2	86.8
P6	560	62.1	14.8
N ($n = 30$)		18.7 (2.2)	
Omissions			
P1	1620	13	4
P2	1980	14	7
P3	1380	11	3
P4	1460	8	1
P5	960	6	2
P6	560	5	0
N ($n = 30$)		0	
Scanning task			
ST (sec)		44.6 (28.6–62.8)	31.3 (20.9–39.7)
FIX		75 (56–123)	55 (39–78)
FIXr (%)		49.5 (33–79)	33.5 (28–61)
FD (sec)		0.42 (0.30–0.52)	0.33 (0.26–0.36)
A (°)		5.0 (4.3–7.2)	5.5 (4.6–7.6)
Dots reported		9 (3–18)	17 (14–20)
N (ST; $n = 30$)		9.3 (0.8)	

Search task: 15 targets, 5 distractors; Scanning task: 20 dots. N: normal control subjects; ST: scanning time; FIX: number of fixations; FIXr: rate of fixation repetitions; FD: fixation duration; A: saccadic amplitude. Numbers refer to means and ranges (in brackets). Dots: number of dots reported.

P2 = 0.33; after practice: P1 = 0.50, P2 = 0.70). However, it should be mentioned that contrast sensitivity was still reduced in both patients when compared with the sensitivity in normal control subjects (cf. Fig. 3.1, p. 93). In the third patient (P3) no such improvement and no change in visual acuity was found.

Finally we also tried to improve reading capacity at least in two cases who now showed Snellen acuity of 0.33 and 0.70 (P4 and P6 in Table 7.1). We started practice with tachistoscopically presenting single words of different length (2–5 letter words; see p. 81), and continued with reading of text material in larger print (Univers, 16 pt). After 62 sessions for P4 and 36 sessions for P6 we found a remarkable improvement in the ability to read for both patients (Table 7.7). Furthermore, both patients had regained, to some extent, the typical staircase

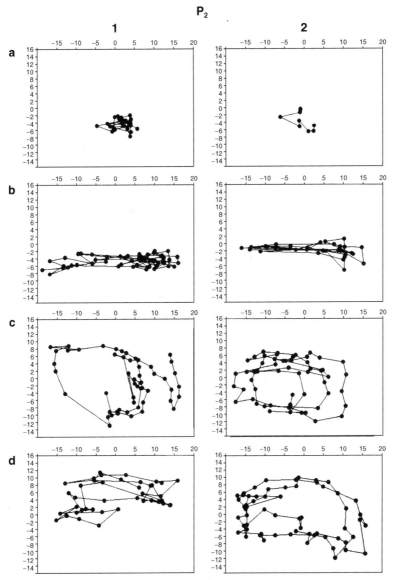

FIG. 7.4 Oculomotor scanning patterns before (1) and after (2) practice with oculomotor scanning in a patient with central scotoma (P2 in Fig. 7.1). a: Fixation (centre; 30sec), b: voluntary horizontal saccades (20°; 30sec), c: scanning of the dot pattern, d: scanning of a scene (Fig. 6.1b). The patient reported 15 out of 20 dots (c) before and 21 dots after practice; he reported 4 out of 7 items (d) before and 6 items after practice. Scanning times (in seconds): 1: c: 37.4, 2: c: 35.9; 1: d: 24.8. 2: d: 42.3. Note the improvement in fixation and visual guidance of saccades (a, b) and the increase in scanning time after practice, which was associated with reporting more visual details. For further details, see Fig. 7.2.

159

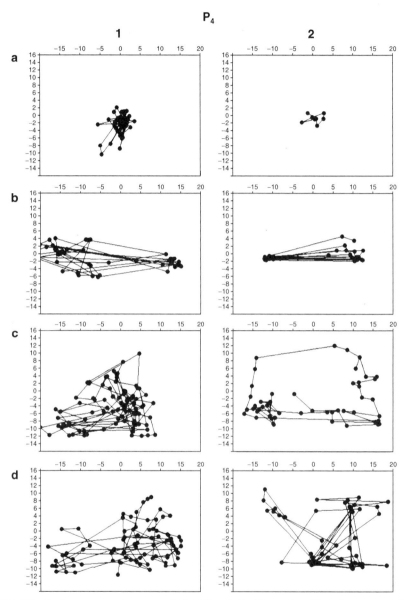

P₄

FIG. 7.5   Oculomotor scanning patterns before (1) and after (2) practice with oculomotor scanning in a patient with central scotoma (P4 in Fig. 7.1). a: Fixation (centre; 30 sec), b: voluntary horizontal saccades (20°; 30sec), c: scanning of the dot pattern, d: scanning of a scene (Fig. 6.1b). The patient reported 10 out of 20 dots (c) before and 16 dots after practice; he reported 3 out of 7 items (d) before and 5 items after practice. Scanning times (in seconds): 1: c: 44.9, 2: c: 36.0; 1: d: 37.5. 2: d: 30.1. Note the improvement in fixation and visual guidance of saccades (a, b) and the improved report of visual details despite decreased scanning time after practice. For further details, see Fig. 7.2.

TABLE 7.6

Acuity and form vision and object recognition in 6 patients with central scotoma before and after treatment. Acuity is expressed in binocular Snellen fractions; visual identification performance is shown in percentage correct responses ($n = 30$/condition; cf. Table 7.3). In P6, acuity was improved after specific practice with reading

	P1	P2	P3	P4	P5	P6
Acuity						
before	0.05	–	0.05	0.05	–	0.22
after	0.29	0.22	0.08	0.33	0.07	0.33
Forms						
before	6.7	3.3	6.7	3.3	0.0	26.7
after	73.3	70.0	53.3	76.7	20.0	100
Fruit						
before	13.3	6.7	6.7	10.0	3.3	53.3
after	70.0	53.3	43.3	90.0	20.0	100
Tools						
before	6.7	3.3	3.3	6.7	0.0	30.0
after	46.7	40.0	30.0	86.7	23.3	93.3
Faces						
before	0.0	6.7	0.0	3.3	0.0	16.7
after	36.7	30.0	16.7	70.0	13.3	86.7
Letters						
before	3.3	3.3	0.0	3.3	6.7	36.7
after	26.7	23.3	13.3	46.7	10.0	70.0

TABLE 7.7

Practice with reading in two patients with central scotoma (P4 and P6 in Fig. 7.1): Procedure and outcome

	No. of trials		Results			
			P4		P6	
	P4	P6	Before	After	Before	After
Procedure						
Reading of single words, ranging from						
2–5 letters; tachistoscopic presentation	2440	840				
Reading of text material (short sentences and						
normal text; Univers 16pt, 30min each)	62	36				
Reading performance (wpm)			3	77	12	98
Normals (n = 25)			174 (138–237)			

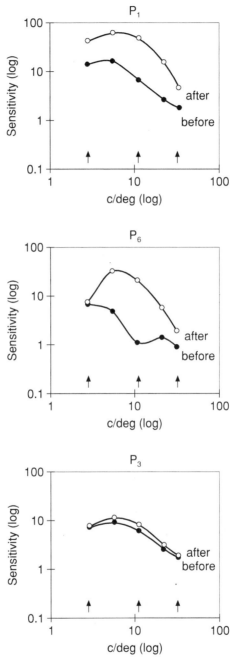

FIG. 7.6 Binocular contrast sensitivity before and after practice in three patients with central scotoma (P1, P3, and P6 in Fig. 7.1). Note improvement in contrast sensitivity in P1 (after 1080 trials) and in P6 (after 2320 trials), but not in P3 despite a higher number of trials (3640). For corresponding data in normal control subjects, see Fig. 3.1, p. 93.

pattern in reading (Fig. 7.7), although speed of reading was still considerably reduced, especially in P4.

Concerning the effect of functional improvement on the remediation of visual disability in everyday life, patients with central scotoma benefited less than did the other groups with homonymous visual field loss. As Table 7.8 shows, the

TABLE 7.8
Reports of six patients with central scotoma about visual difficulties in everyday life before and after treatment

	No. of patients	
Difficulties	Before	After
Visual orientation in familiar surroundings	6	2
Visual orientation in unfamiliar surroundings	6	4
Bumping against obstacles	5	4
Visual identification of objects and scenes	6	3
Visual identification of faces	6	3
Visual recognition of familiar faces	6	4
Reading	6	4

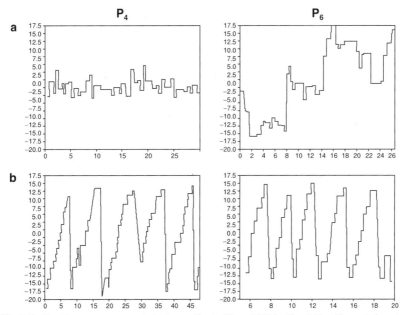

FIG. 7.7   Reading eye movements in two patients (P4 and P6 in Fig. 7.1) with central scotoma before (a) and after (b) practice. Note improvement in the pattern of reading eye movements after practice. x-axis: time period of recording (in seconds), y-axis: horizontal extension of line (in degress). 0 = centre, negative values left, positive values right.

benefit was mainly achieved in familiar surroundings, but even there the patients still had difficulties in finding objects, for example a chair, a knife, a fork, or a spoon, a cup or a glass on a dining table, clothes in the wardrobe, toilet requisites in the bathroom, the partner among friends, etc. Nevertheless all but two patients reported a distinct reduction of their visual disabilities.

In conclusion, patients with central scotoma can also benefit from systematic practice of searching and oculomotor scanning; some of them also showed an increase in visual acuity. It is, however, only fair to state that the improvement was of limited impact for the reduction of patients' visual disabilities, and that the treatment was a difficult, time-consuming, and all too often frustrating task for both the patient and the therapist. Whether this is due to the fact that this group of patients has only a minor chance of recovery, or whether we need more special methods of practice cannot be answered with certainty at present. Possibly, both arguments hold true. Even then one should be encouraged to risk further attempts to remediate the severe visual disabilities of these patients.

References

Acheson, J.F., & Sanders, M.D. (1995). Vision. *Journal of Neurology, Neurosurgery, and Psychiatry, 59*, 4–15.

Adler, A. (1944). Disintegration and restoration of optic recognition in visual agnosia. *Archives of Neurology and Psychiatry, 51*, 243–259.

Adler, A. (1950). Course and outcome of visual agnosia. *Journal of Nervous and Mental Diseases, 3*, 41–51.

Albert, M.L., Reches, A., & Silverberg, R. (1975). Hemianopic colour blindness. *Journal of Neurology, Neurosurgery, and Psychiatry, 38*, 546–549.

Aldrich, M.S., Alessi, A.G., Beck, R.W., & Gilman, S. (1987). Cortical blindness: Etiology, diagnosis, and prognosis. *Annals of Neurology, 21*, 149–158.

Alexander, M.P., & Albert, M.L. (1983). The anatomical basis of visual agnosia. In A. Kertesz (Ed.), *Localization in Neuropsychology* (pp. 393–415). New York: Academic Press.

Allison, R.S., Hurwitz, L.J., White, G.J., & Wilmot, T.J. (1969). A follow-up study of a patient with Balint's syndrome. *Neuropsychologia, 7*, 319–333.

Anderson, S.W., & Rizzo, M. (1995). Recovery and rehabilitation of visual cortical dysfunction. *NeuroRehabilitation, 5*, 129–140.

Anstis, S.M. (1974). A chart demonstrating variations in acuity with retinal position. *Vision Research, 14*, 579–582.

Antonucci, G., Guariglia, C., Judica, A., Magnotti, L., Paolucci, S., Pizzamiglio, L., & Zoccolotti, P. (1995). Effectiveness of neglect rehabilitation in a randomized group study. *Journal of Clinical and Experimental Neuropsychology, 17*, 383–389.

Arden, G.B. (1978). The importance of measuring contrast sensitivity in cases with visual disturbance. *British Journal of Ophthalmology, 62*, 198–209.

Aulhorn, E., & Harms, H. (1972). Visual perimetry. In D. Jameson & L.M. Hurvich (Eds), *Visual Psychophysics. Handbook of Sensory Physiology* VII/4 (pp. 102–144). Berlin: Springer.

Baddeley, A., Meade, T., & Newcombe, F. (1980). Design problems in research on rehabilitation after brain damage. *International Rehabilitation Medicine, 2*, 138–142.

Balint, R. (1909). Seelenlähmung des "Schauens", optische Ataxie, räumliche Störung der Aufmerksamkeit. *Monatsschrift für Psychiatrie und Neurologie, 25*, 51–81.

Balliet, R., Blood, K.M.T., & Bach-y-Rita, P. (1985). Visual field rehabilitation in the cortically blind? *Journal of Neurology, Neurosurgery, and Psychiatry, 48*, 1113–1124.

Barlow, D.H., & Hersen, M. (1985). *Single case experimental design: Strategies for studying behaviour change.* (2nd ed.). New York: Pergamon.

Benton, A.L., & Tranel, D. (1993). Visuoperceptual, visuospatial, and visuoconstructive disorders. In K.M. Heilman & E. Valenstein (Eds), *Clinical Neuropsychology,* (3rd ed.). (pp. 165–213). New York: Oxford University Press.

Bergman, P.S. (1957). Cerebral blindness. *Archives of Neurology and Psychiatry, 78,* 568–584.

Bodis-Wollner, I. (1972). Visual acuity and contrast sensitivity in patients with cerebral lesions. *Science, 178,* 769–771.

Bodis-Wollner, I. (1976). Vulnerability of spatial frequency channels in cerebral lesions. *Nature, 261,* 309–311.

Bodis-Wollner, I., & Diamond, S.P. (1976). The measurement of spatial contrast sensitivity in cases of blurred vision associated with cerebral lesions. *Brain, 99,* 695–710.

Bosley, T.M., Dann, R., Silver, F.L., Alavi, A., Kushner, M., Chawluk, J.B., Savino, P.J., Sergott, R.C., Schatz, N.J., & Raivich, M. (1987). Recovery of vision after ischemic lesions: Positron emission tomography. *Annals of Neurology, 21,* 444–450.

Bruyer, R., Laterre, C., Seron, F.X., Feyereisen, P. Strypsetin, E. Pierrard, E., & Rectem, D. (1983). A case of prosopagnosia with some preserved covert remembrance of familiar faces. *Brain and Cognition, 2,* 257–284.

Bulens, C., Meerwaldt, J.D., van der Wildt, G.J., & Kemink, D. (1989). Spatial contrast sensitivity in unilateral cerebral ischemic lesions involving the posterior visual pathway. *Brain, 112,* 507–520.

Calabria, G., Gandolfo, E., Rolando, M., Capris, P., & Burtolo, C. (1985). Ergoperimetry in patients with severe visual field damage. In A. Heijl & E.L. Greve (Eds), *Proceedings of the 6th International Visual Field Symposium* (pp. 349–352). Dordrecht: Dr. W. Junk Publishers.

Celesia, G.G., Brigell, M.G., & Vaphiades, M.S. (1997). Hemianopic anosognosia. *Neurology, 49,* 88–97.

Charnallet, A., Rousset, S., Carbonnel, S., & Pellat, J. (1996). A case study of a strong perceptual deficit without agnosia—evidence against sequential perception and memory. *Brain & Cognition, 32,* 115–117.

Chedru, F., Leblanc, M., & Lhermitte, ·F. (1973). Visual searching in normal and brain-damaged subjects. *Cortex, 9,* 94–111.

Chelazzi, L., Miller, E.K., Duncan, J., & Desimone, R. (1993). A neural basis of visual search in inferotemporal cortex. *Nature, 363,* 345–347.

Ciuffreda, K.J., Kenyon, R.V., & Stark, L. (1985). Eye movements during reading: Further case reports. *American Journal of Optometry and Physiological Optics, 62,* 844–852.

Corbetta, M., Miezin, F.M., Shulman, G.L., & Petersen, S.E. (1993). A PET study of visual spatial attention. *Journal of Neuroscience, 13,* 1202–1226.

Courtney, A.J., & Shou, C.H. (1985). Simple measures of visual-lobe size and search performance. *Ergonomics, 28,* 1319–1331.

Cowey, A. (1967). Perimetric study of visual field defects in monkeys after cortical and retinal ablations. *Quarterly Journal of Experimental Psychology, 19,* 232–245.

Cowey, A. (1994). Cortical visual areas and the neurobiology of higher visual processes. In M.J. Farah & G. Ratcliff (Eds), *The Neuropsychology of High-Level Vision* (pp. 3–31). Hillsdale, NJ: Erlbaum.

Critchley, M. (1949). The problem of awareness or non-awareness of hemianopic field defects. *Transactions of the Ophthalmological Society UK, 69,* 95–109.

Damasio, A.R., Tranel, D., & Damasio, H. (1989). Disorders of visual recognition. In F. Boller & J. Grafman (Eds), *Handbook of Neuropsychology,* (Vol. 2, pp. 317–322). Amsterdam: Elsevier Science Publishers Biomedical Division.

Damasio, A.R., Yamada, T., Damasio, H., Corbett, J., & McKee, J. (1980). Central achromatopsia: Behavioral, anatomic, physiological aspects. *Neurology, 30,* 1064–1071.

De Haan, E.H., Heywood, C.A., Young, A.W., Edelstyn, N., & Newcombe, F. (1995). Ettlinger revisited: The relation between agnosia and sensory impairment. *Journal of Neurology, Neurosurgery, and Psychiatry*, *58*, 350–356.

De Renzi, E. (1982). *Disorders of space exploration and cognition*. Chichester, New York: Wiley.

Desimone, R., & Ungerleider, L.G. (1989). Neural mechanisms of visual processing in monkeys. In F. Boller & J. Grafman (Eds), *Handbook of neuropsychology*, (Vol. 2, pp. 267–299). Amsterdam: Elsevier.

Diller, L., Ben-Yishay, Y., Gerstman, J.L., Goodkin, R., & Gordon, W. (1974). *Studies in cognition and rehabilitation in hemiplegia. Rehabilitation monograph No. 50*. New York Institute of Rehabilitation Medicine, New York.

Driver, J., & Mattingley, J.B. (1995). Selective attention in humans: Normality and pathology. *Current Opinion in Neurobiology*, *5*, 191–197.

Dromerick, A.W., & Reding, M.J. (1995). Functional outcome for patients with hemiparesis, hemihypaesthesia, and hemianopsia. Does lesion location matter? *Stroke*, *26*, 2023–2026.

Eber, A.M., Metz-Lutz, M.N., Strubel, D., Vetrano, E., & Collard, M. (1988). Electro-oculographic study of reading in hemianopic patients. *Revue Neurologique*, *144*, 515–518.

Ellenberger, C.Jr. (1974). Modern perimetry in neuro-ophthalmic diagnosis. *Archives of Neurology*, *30*, 193–201.

Farnsworth, D. (1943). The Farnsworth–Munsell 100-hue and dichotomous tests for colour vision. *Journal of the Optical Society of America*, *33*, 569–578.

Feibel, J.H., & Springer, C.J. (1982). Depression and failure to resume social activities after stroke. *Archives of Physical Medicine and Medical Rehabilitation*, *63*, 276–278.

Fellemann, D.J., & van Essen, D.C. (1991). Distributed hierarchical processing in the primate cerebral cortex. *Cerebral Cortex*, *1*, 1–47.

Fiorentini, A., & Berardi, N. (1980). Perceptual learning specific for orientation and spatial frequency. *Nature*, *287*, 43–44.

Frisén, L. (1980). The neurology of visual acuity. *Brain*, *103*, 639–670.

Frommer, G.P. (1978). Subtotal lesions: Implications for coding and recovery of function. In S. Finger (Ed.) *Recovery from brain damage: Research and theory* (pp. 217–280). New York: Plenum Press.

Gainotti, G., Silveri, M.C., Daniele, A., & Giustolisi, L. (1995). Neuroanatomical correlates of category-specific semantic disorders: A critical survey. *Memory*, *3*, 247–264.

Gassel, M.M., & Williams, D. (1963a). Visual functions in patients with homonymous hemianopia. Part II. Oculomotor mechanisms. *Brain*, *86*, 1–36.

Gassel, M.M., & Williams, D. (1963b). Visual functions in patients with homonymous hemianopia. Part III. The completion phenomenon; insight and attitude to the defect; and visual functional efficiency. *Brain*, *86*, 229–260.

Gianutsos, R., & Matheson, P. (1987). The rehabilitation of visual perceptual disorders attributable to brain injury. In: M.J. Meier, A.L. Benton & L. Diller (Eds), *Neuropsychological rehabilitation* (pp. 202–241). Edinburgh: Churchill Livingstone.

Gloning, I., Gloning, K., & Hoff, H. (1968). *Neuropsychological symptoms and syndromes in lesions of the occipital lobe and adjacent areas*. Paris: Gauthier-Villar.

Gloning, I., Gloning, K., & Tschabitscher, H. (1962). Die occipitale Blindheit auf vaskulärer Basis. *Von Graefes Archiv für Ophthalmologie*, *165*, 138–177.

Goto, K., Tagawa, K., Uemura, K., Ishii, K., & Takahashi, S. (1979). Posterior cerebral artery occlusion: Clinical, computed tomographic, and angiographic correlation. *Radiology*, *132*, 357–368.

Groswasser, Z., Cohen, M., & Blankstein, E. (1990). Polytrauma associated with traumatic brain injury: Incidence, nature and impact on rehabilitation outcome. *Brain Injury*, *4*, 161–166.

Grüsser, O.-J., & Landis, T. (1991). *Visual agnosias and other disturbances of visual perception and cognition*. Boca Raton: CRC Press.

Halligan, P.W., Cockburn, J., & Wilson, B.A. (1991). The behavioral assessment of neglect. *Neuropsychological Rehabilitation, 1,* 5–32.

Harrington, D.O. (1976). *The Visual Fields.* (4th ed.). St. Louis: Mosby.

Hecaen, H., & Ajuriaguerra, J. de (1954). Balint's syndrome (psychic paralysis of fixation) and its minor forms. *Brain, 77,* 373–400.

Henderson, V.W. (1982). Impaired hue discrimination in homonymous visual fields. *Archives of Neurology, 39,* 418–419.

Hess, R.F. (1984). On the assessment of contrast threshold functions for anomalous vision. *British Orthoptic Journal, 41,* 1–14.

Hess, R.F., Zihl, J., Pointer, S.J., & Schmid, Ch. (1990). The contrast sensitivity deficit in cases with cerebral lesions. *Clinical Vision Sciences, 5,* 203–215.

Heywood, C.A., Gadotti, A., & Cowey, A. (1992). Cortical area V4 and its role in the perception of color. *The Journal of Neuroscience, 12,* 4056–4065.

Heywood, C.A., Wilson, B., & Cowey, A. (1987). A case study of cortical colour blindness with relatively intact achromatic discrimination. *Journal of Neurology, Neurosurgery, and Psychiatry, 50,* 22–29.

Hier, D.B., Mondlock, J., & Caplan, L.R. (1983a). Behavioral abnormalities after right hemisphere stroke. *Neurology, 33,* 337–344.

Hier, D.B., Mondlock, J., & Caplan, L.R. (1983b). Recovery of behavioral abnormalities after right hemisphere stroke. *Neurology, 33,* 345–350.

Hillis, E.H., & Caramazza, A. (1992). The reading process and its disorders. In D.I. Margolin (Ed.), *Cognitive neuropsychology in clinical practice* (pp. 229–262). New York, Oxford: Oxford University Press.

Humphrey, N.K. (1974). Vision in a monkey without striate cortex: A case study. *Perception, 3,* 241–255.

Humphreys, G.W., & Riddoch, M.J. (1994). Visual object processing in normality and pathology: Implications for rehabilitation. In M.J. Riddoch & G.W. Humphreys (Eds), *Cognitive neuropsychology and cognitive rehabilitation* (pp. 39–76). Hove, UK: Lawrence Erlbaum Associates Ltd.

Humphreys, G.W., Riddoch, M.J., & Wallesch, C.-W. (1996). Poppelreuter's case of Merk: The analysis of visual disturbances following a gunshot wound to the brain. In: C. Code, C.-W. Wallesch, Y. Joanette & A. Rosch (Eds), *Classical cases in neuropsychology* (pp. 77–88). Hove, UK: Psychology Press.

Igersheimer, J. (1919). Zur Pathologie der Sehbahn. IV. Gesichtsfeldverbesserung bei Hemianopikern. *Albrecht von Grefes Archiv für Ophthalmologie, 100,* 357–369.

Ikeda, M., & Saida, S. (1978). Span of recognition in reading. *Vision Research, 18,* 83–88.

Inhoff, A.W. (1987). Parafoveal word perception during eye fixations in reading: Effects of visual salience and word structure. In M. Coltheart (Ed.), *Attention and performance XII: The psychology of reading* (pp. 403–418). Hove, UK: Lawrence Erlbaum Associates Ltd.

Ishiai, S., Furukawa, T., & Tsukagoshi, H. (1987). Eye-fixation patterns in homonymous hemianopia and unilateral spatial neglect. *Neuropsychologia, 25,* 675–679.

Jackowski, M.M., Sturr, J.F., Taub, H.A., & Turk, M.A. (1996). Photophobia in patients with traumatic brain injury: Uses of light-filtering lenses to enhance contrast sensitivity and reading rate. *NeuroRehabilitation, 6,* 193–201.

Kasten, E., & Sabel, B.A. (1995). Visual field enlargement after computer training in brain-damaged patients with homonymous deficits—an open pilot trial. *Restorative Neurology & Neuroscience, 8,* 113–127.

Kerkhoff, G. (1988). Visuelle Raumwahrnehmung und Raumoperationen. In D. von Cramon & J. Zihl (Eds). *Neuropsychologische Rehabilitation* (pp. 197–214). Berlin: Springer.

Kerkhoff, G., Münssinger, U., Eberle-Strauss, G., & Stögerer, E. (1992a). Rehabilitation of hemianopic alexia in patients with postgeniculate visual field disorders. *Neuropsychological Rehabilitation, 2,* 21–42.

Kerkhoff, G., Münssinger, U., Haaf, E., Eberle-Strauss, G., & Stögerer, E. (1992b). Rehabilitation of homonymous scotomata in patients with postgeniculate damage of the visual system: Saccadic compensation training. *Restorative Neurology and Neuroscience, 4,* 245–254.

Kerkhoff, G., Münssinger, U., & Meier, E. (1994). Neurovisual rehabilitation in cerebral blindness. *Archives of Neurology, 51,* 474–481.

Kerkhoff, G., Schaub, J., & Zihl, J. (1990). Assessment of cerebral visual disorders by patient-questionnaire. [In German]. *Nervenarzt, 61,* 711–718.

Kertesz, A. (1979). Visual agnosia: The dual deficit of perception and recognition. *Cortex, 15,* 403–419.

Klüver, H. (1942). Functional significance of the geniculo-striate system. *Biological Symposia, 7,* 253–299.

Koehler, P.J., Endtz, L.J., Te Velde, J., & Hekster, R.E. (1986). Aware or non-aware. On the significance of awareness for the localization of the lesion responsible for homonymous hemianopia. *Journal of Neurological Sciences, 75,* 255–262.

Kustov, A.A., & Robinson, D.L. (1996). Shared neural control of attentional shifts and eye movements. *Nature, 384,* 74–77.

Legge, D.E., Pelli, D.G., Rubin, G.S., & Schleske, M.M. (1985). Psychophysics of reading. I. Normal vision. *Vision Research, 25,* 239–252.

Leigh, R.J., & Zee D.S. (1991). *The neurology of eye movements.* (2nd ed.). Philadelphia: F.A. Davis.

Levine, D.N. (1990). Unawareness of visual and sensorimotor defects: A hypothesis. *Brain and Cognition, 13,* 231–281.

Lezak, M.D. (1995). *Neuropsychological assessment.* (3rd ed.). New York, Oxford: Oxford University Press.

Liepmann, H., & Kalmus, E. (1900). Über eine Augenmaassstörung bei Hemianopikern. *Berliner Klinische Wochenschrift, 38,* 838–842.

Lissauer, H. (1890). Ein Fall von Seelenblindheit nebst einem Beitrage zur Theorie derselben. *Archiv für Psychiatrie und Nervenkrankheiten, 21,* 222–270.

Lovie-Kitchin, J., Mainstone, J., Robinson, J., & Brown, P. (1990). What areas of the visual field are important for mobility in low vision patients? *Clinical Vision Sciences, 5,* 249–263.

Lütgehetmann, R., & Stäbler, M. (1992). Deficiencies of visual spatial orientation: Diagnostic and therapy of brain-damaged patients [in German]. *Zeitschrift für Neuropsychologie, 3,* 130–142.

Mackensen, G. (1962). Die Untersuchung der Lesefähigkeit als klinische Funktionsprüfung. *Fortschritte der Augenheilkunde, 12,* 344–379.

McCarthy, R.A., & Warrington, E.K. (1988). Evidence for modality-specific meaning systems in the brain. *Nature, 334,* 428–430.

McConkie, G.W., & Rayner, K. (1975). The span of the effective stimulus during a fixation in reading. *Perception & Psychophysics, 17,* 578–586.

McConkie, G.W., & Rayner, K. (1976). Asymmetry of the perceptual span in reading. *Bulletin of the Psychonomic Society, 8,* 365–368.

McDonald, W.I., & Barnes, D. (1992). The ocular manifestations of multiple sclerosis. 1. Abnormalities of the afferent visual system. *Journal of Neurology, Neurosurgery, and Psychiatry, 55,* 747–752.

Meadows, J.C. (1974). Disturbed perception of colours associated with localized cerebral lesions. *Brain, 97,* 615–632.

Meerwaldt, J.D. (1983). Spatial disorientation in right-hemisphere infarction: A study of the speed of recovery. *Journal of Neurology, Neurosurgery, and Psychiatry, 46,* 426–429.

Meerwaldt, J.D., & van Harskamp, F. (1982). Spatial disorientation in right-hemisphere infarction. *Journal of Neurology, Neurosurgery, and Psychiatry, 45,* 586–590.

Meienberg, O., Zangemeister, E.H., Rosenberg, M., Hoyt, W.F., & Stark, L. (1981). Saccadic eye movements strategies in patients with homonymous hemianopia. *Annals of Neurology, 9,* 537–544.

Mesulam, M.M. (1981). A cortical network for directed visual attention and unilateral neglect. *Annals of Neurology, 10,* 309–325.

Miller, N.R. (1982). Topical diagnosis of retrochiasmal visual field defects. In *Clinical Neuro-ophthalmology*, (Vol. 1, pp. 127–147). Baltimore: Williams & Wilkins.

Milner, A.D., Perrett, D.I., Johnston, R.S., Benson, P.J., Jordan, T.R., Heeley, D.W., Betucci, D., Mortara, F., Mutani, R., Terazzi, E., & Davidson, D.L.W. (1991). Perception and action in "Visual form agnosia". *Brain, 114,* 405–428.

Mohler, C.W., & Wurtz, R.H. (1977). Role of striate cortex and superior colliculus in visual guidance of saccadic eye movements. *Journal of Neurophysiology, 40,* 74–94.

Montero, J., Pena, J., Genis, D., Rubio, F., Peres-Serra, J., & Barraquer-Bordas, L. (1982). Balint's syndrome. *Acta Neurologica Belgica, 82,* 270–280.

Morel, A., & Bullier, J. (1990). Anatomical segregation of two cortical visual pathways in the macaque monkey. *Visual Neuroscience, 4,* 555–578.

Munsell Book of Color (1976). Baltimore (MD): MacBeth Division of Kollmorgen Corporation.

Ogden, J.A. (1993). Visual object agnosia, prosopagnosia, achromatopsia, loss of visual imagery, and autobiographical amnesia following recovery from cortical blindness: Case M.H. *Neuropsychologia, 31,* 571–589.

Pearlman, A.L., Birch, J., & Meadows, J.C. (1979). Cerebral colour blindness: An acquired defect in hue discrimination. *Annals of Neurology, 5,* 253–261.

Petersen, S.E., Robinson, D.L., & Morris, J.D. (1987). Contributions of the pulvinar to visual spatial attention. *Neuropsychologia, 25,* 97–105.

Pierrot-Deseilligny, C., Gray, F., & Brunet, P. (1986). Infarcts of both inferior parietal lobules with impairment of visually guided eye movements, peripheral visual inattention and optic apraxia. *Brain, 109,* 81–97.

Pierrot-Deseilligny, Ch., Rivaud, S., Gaymard, B. Müri, R., & Vermersch, A.I. (1995). Cortical control of saccades. *Annals of Neurology, 37,* 557–567.

Pizzamiglio, L., Antonucci, G., Guariglia, C., Judica, A., Montenero, P., Razzano, C., & Zoccolotti, P. (1992). Cognitive rehabilitation of the hemineglect disorders in chronic patients with unilateral right brain damage. *Journal of Clinical and Experimental Neuropsychology, 14,* 901–923.

Plant, G.T., Kermode, A.G., Turano, G., Moseley, I.F., Miller, D.H., MacManus, D.G., Halliday, A.M., & McDonald, W.I. (1992). Symptomatic retrochiasmal lesions in multiple sclerosis: Clinical features, visual evoked potentials, and magnetic resonance imaging. *Neurology, 42,* 68–76.

Pommerenke, K., & Markowitsch, J.H. (1989). Rehabilitation training of homonymous visual field defects in patients with postgeniculate damage to the visual system. *Restorative Neurology & Neurosciences, 1,* 47–63.

Pöppel, E. (1986). Long-range colour-generating interactions across the retina. *Nature, 320,* 523–525.

Pöppel, E., Brinkmann, R., von Cramon, D., & Singer, W. (1978). Association and dissociation of visual functions in a case of bilateral occipital lobe infarction. *Archiv für Psychiatrie und Nervenkrankheiten, 225,* 1–21.

Poppelreuter, W. (1917/1990). *Disturbances of lower and higher visual capacities caused by occipital damage.* Transl. J. Zihl & L. Weiskrantz. Oxford: Oxford University Press (Clarendon).

Poulson, H.L., Galetta, S.L., Grossman, M., & Alavi, A. (1994). Hemiachromatopsia after occipitotemporal infarcts. *American Journal of Ophthalmology, 118,* 518–523.

Powell, J., & Davidoff, D. (1995). Selective impairments of object knowledge in a case of acquired cortical blindness. *Memory, 3,* 435–461.

Raymond, M.J., Bennett, T.L., Malia, K.B., & Bewick K.C. (1996). Rehabilitation of visual processing deficits following brain injury. *NeuroRehabilitation, 6,* 229–240.

Rayner, K., McConkie, G.W., & Ehrlich, S. (1978). Eye movements and integration of information across fixations. *Journal of Experimental Psychology: Human Perception & Performance, 4,* 529–544.

Rayner, K., & Pollatsek, A. (1987). Eye movements in reading: A tutorial review. In M. Coltheart (Ed.), *Attention and performance XII: The psychology of reading* (pp. 327–362). Hove, UK: Lawrence Erlbaum Associates Ltd.

Reding, M.J., & Potes, E. (1988). Rehabilitation outcome following initial unilateral hemispheric stroke: Life table analysis approach. *Stroke, 19*, 1354–1358.

Richards, P.M., & Ruff, R.M. (1989). Motivational effects on neuropsychological functioning: comparison of depressed versus nondepressed individuals. *Journal of Consulting and Clinical Psychology, 57*, 396–402.

Rizzo, M., Smith, V., Pokorny, J., & Damasio, A.R. (1993). Colour perception profiles in central achromatopsia. *Neurology, 43*, 995–1001.

Robertson, L.C. (1992). Perceptual organization and attentional search in cognitive deficits. In D.I. Margolin (Ed.), *Cognitive neuropsychology in clinical practice* (pp. 70–95). New York, Oxford: Oxford University Press.

Robertson, I.H. (1994). Methodology in neuropsychological rehabilitation research. *Neuropsychological Rehabilitation, 4*, 1–6.

Robinson, D.L. (1993). Functional contributions of the primate pulvinar. *Progress in Brain Research, 95*, 371–380.

Robinson, D.L., & Petersen, S.E. (1992). The pulvinar and visual salience. *Trends in Neurosciences, 15*, 127–132.

Rockland, K.S., & Pandya, D.N. (1981). Cortical connections of the occipital lobe in the rhesus monkey: Interconnections between areas 17, 18, 19 and the superior temporal sulcus. *Brain Research, 212*, 249–270.

Rossi, P.W., Kheyfets, S., & Reding, M. (1990). Fresnal lenses improve visual perception in stroke patients with homonymous hemianopia or unilateral visual neglect. *Neurology, 40*, 1587–1599.

Rothi, L.J., & Horner, J. (1983). Restitution and substitution: Two theories of recovery with application to neurobehavioral treatment. *Journal of Clinical Neuropsychology, 5*, 73–81.

Sarno, J.E., & Sarno, M.T. (1979). *Stroke: A guide for patients and their families*. New York: McGraw Hill.

Savino, P.J., Paris, M., Schatz, N.J., & Corbett, J.J. (1978). Optic tract syndrome. *Archives of Ophthalmology, 96*, 656–663.

Sekuler, R., & Blake, R. (1985). *Perception*. New York: Alfred A. Knopf.

Selemon, L.D., & Goldman-Rakic, P.S. (1988). Common cortical and subcortical targets of the dorsolateral prefrontal and posterior parietal cortices in the rhesus monkey: Evidence for a distributed neural network subserving spatially guided behavior. *Journal of Neuroscience, 8*, 4049–4068.

Seltzer, B., & Pandya, D.N. (1984). Further observations on parieto-temporal connections in the rhesus monkey. *Experimental Brain Research, 55*, 301–312.

Sergent, J. (1988). An investigation into perceptual completion in blind areas of the visual field. *Brain, 111*, 347–373.

Shipp, S., de Jong, B.M., Zihl, J., Frackowiak, R.S.J., & Zeki, S. (1994). The brain activity related to residual motion vision in a patient with bilateral lesions to V5. *Brain, 117*, 1023–1038.

Sidman, M., & Stoddard, L.T. (1967). The effectiveness of fading in programming a simultaneous form discrimination for retarded children. *Journal of the Experimental Analysis of Behavior, 10*, 3–15.

Siemerling, E. (1890). Ein Fall von sogenannter Seelenblindheit nebst anderweitigen cerebralen Symptomen. *Archiv für Psychiatrie und Nervenkrankheiten, 21*, 284–289.

Singer, W. (1979). Central core control of visual-cortex functions. In F.O. Schmitt & F.G. Worden (Eds), *The neuroscienes fourth study program* (pp. 1093–1110). Cambridge, MA, and London: MIT Press.

Slamovits, T.L., Rosen, C.E., Cheng, K.P., & Striph, G.G. (1991). Visual recovery in patients with optic neuritis and visual loss to no light perception. *American Journal of Ophthalmology, 111*, 209–214.

Sloan, L.L. (1971). The Tübingen perimeter of Aulhorn and Harms. *Archives of Ophthalmology*, *86*, 612–622.

Small, S.L., Hart, J., Nguyen, T., & Gordon, B. (1995). Distributed representations of semantic knowledge in the brain. *Brain, 118*, 441–453.

Sparr, S.A., Jay, M., Drislane, F.W., & Venna, N. (1991). A historic case of visual agnosia revisited after 40 years. *Brain, 114*, 789–800.

Stein, D.G. (1994). Brain damage and recovery. *Progress in Brain Research, 100*, 203–211.

Symonds, C., & MacKenzie, I. (1957). Bilateral loss of vision from cerebral infarction. *Brain, 80*, 415–455.

Teuber, H.-L. (1975). Recovery of function after brain injury in man. In *Outcome of severe damage to the central nervous system* (pp. 159–190). Ciba Foundation Symposium 34 (New Series). Amsterdam: Elsevier.

Teuber, H.-L., Battersby, W.S., & Bender, M.B. (1960). *Visual field defects after penetrating missile wounds of the brain*. Cambridge, MA: Harvard University Press.

Tootell, R.B.H., Dale, A.M., Sereno, M.I., & Malach, R. (1996). New images from human visual cortex. *Trends in Neurosciences, 19*, 481–489.

Traccis, S., Puliga, M.V., Ruiu, M.C., Marras, M.A., & Rosati, G. (1991). Unilateral occipital lesion causing hemianopia affects the acoustic saccadic programming. *Neurology, 41*, 1633–1638.

Trobe, J.D., Lorber, M.L., & Schlezinger, N.S. (1973). Isolated homonymous hemianopia. *Archives of Ophthalmology, 89*, 377–381.

Uemura, T., Arai, Y., & Shimazaki, C. (1980). Eye–head coordination during lateral gaze in normal subjects. *Acta Otolaryngica, 90*, 191–198.

Uzzel, B.P., Dolinskas, C.A., & Langfitt, T.W. (1988). Visual field defects in relation to head injury severity. *Archives of Neurology, 45*, 420–424.

Van der Wildt, G.J., & Bergsma, P.B. (1997). Visual field enlargement by neuropsychological training in a hemianopsia patient. *Documenta Ophthalmologica, 93*, 277–292.

Verriest, G., Bailey, I.L., Calabria, G., Campos, E., Crick, R.P., Enoch, J.M., Esterman, B., Friedman, A.C., Hill, A.R., Ikeda, M., Johnson, C.A., Overington, I., Ronchi, L., Saida, S., Serra, A., Villani, S., Weale, R.A., Wolbarsht, M.L., & Zingirian, M. (1985). The occupational visual field: II. Practical aspects: The functional visual field in abnormal conditions and its relationship to visual ergonomics, visual impairment and job fitness. In A. Heijl & E.L. Greve (Eds), *Proceedings of the 6th International Visual Field Symposium* (pp. 281–326). Dordrecht: Dr. W. Junk Publishers.

Walsh, Th.J. (1985). Blurred vision. In Th.J. Walsh (Ed.), *Neuro-ophthalmology: Clinical signs and symptoms* (pp. 343–385). Philadelphia: Lea & Febiger.

Walsh, F.B., & Hoyt, W.F. (1969). *Clinical Neuro-ophthalmology*. (3rd Ed.). (Vol. 1). Baltimore: Williams & Wilkins.

Wapner, W., Judd, T., & Gardner, H. (1978). Visual agnosia in an artist. *Cortex, 14*, 343–364.

Warrington, E.K. (1985). Agnosia: The impairment of object recognition. In J.A.M. Frederiks (Ed.), *Handbook of Clinical Neurology. Vol 1 (45): Clinical Neuropsychology* (pp. 333–349). Amsterdam: Elsevier.

Weinberg, J., Diller, L., Gordon, W.A., Gerstman, L.J., Lieberman, A., Lakin, P., Hodges, G., & Ezrachi, O. (1979). Training sensory awareness and spatial organisation in people with right brain damage. *Archives of Physical Medicine and Rehabilitation, 60*, 491–496.

Weiss, N. (1969). Management of the low vision patient with peripheral field loss. *Journal of the American Optometric Association, 40*, 830–832.

Weiss, N. (1972). An application of cemented prism with severe field loss. *American Journal of Optometry and Archives of the Academy of Optometrists, 49*, 261–264.

Weiskrantz, L. (1986). *Blindsight—A case study and its implications*. Oxford: Oxford University Press.

Weiskrantz, L., & Cowey, A. (1970). Filling in the scotoma: A study of residual vision after striate cortex lesions in monkeys. In E. Stellar & J.M. Sprague (Eds), *Progress in physiological psychology*, (Vol. 3, pp. 237–260). New York: Academic Press.

Wilbrand, H. (1907). Über die makulär-hemianopische Lesestörung und die von Monakow'sche Projektion der Makula auf die Sehsphäre. *Klinische Monatsblätter für Augenheilkunde, 45*, 1–39.

Wilbrand, H., & Saenger, A. (1917). *Die Neurologie des Auges. Band 7: Die Erkrankungen der Sehbahn vom Tractus bis in den Cortex*. Wiesbaden: J.F. Bergmann.

Williams, D., & Gassel, M.M. (1962). Visual function in patients with homonymous hemianopia. Part I. The visual fields. *Brain, 85*, 175–250.

Wilson, B.A., Baddeley, A. Evans, J., & Shiel, A. (1994). Errorless learning in the rehabilitation of memory impaired people. *Neuropsychological Rehabilitation, 4*, 307–326.

Wilson, B., & Davidoff, J. (1993). Partial recovery from visual object agnosia: A 10 year follow-up study. *Cortex, 29*, 529–542.

Wilson, B.A., & Evans, J.J. (1996). Error-free learning in the rehabilitation of people with memory impairments. *Journal of Head Trauma Rehabilitation, 11*, 54–64.

Young, R.S.L., Fishman, G.A., & Chen, F. (1980). Traumatically acquired color vision defect. *Investigative Ophthalmology & Visual Science, 19*, 545–549.

Young, L.R., & Sheena, D. (1975). Survey of eye movement recording methods. *Behavior Research Methods and Instrumentation, 7*, 397–429.

Zagorski, A. (1867). Ein Fall von gleichseitiger Hemiopie nach apoplectischem Insult mit vollständiger Restitution. *Klinische Monatsblätter für Augenheilkunde, 5*, 322–325.

Zangemeister, W.H., Meienberg, O., Stark, L., & Hoyt, W.F. (1982). Eye-head coordination in homonymous hemianopia. *Journal of Neurology, 226*, 243–254.

Zeki, S.M. (1978). Functional specialisation in the visual cortex of the rhesus monkey. *Nature, 274*, 423–428.

Zeki, S. (1993). *A vision of the brain*. Oxford: Blackwell Scientific.

Zihl, J. (1980). "Blindsight": Improvement of visually guided eye movements by systematic practice in patients with cerebral blindness. *Neuropsychologia, 18*, 71–77.

Zihl, J. (1981). Recovery of visual functions in patients with cerebral blindness. *Experimental Brain Research, 44*, 159–169.

Zihl, J. (1988). Sehen. In D. von Cramon & J. Zihl (Eds), *Neuropsychologische Rehabilitation* (pp. 105–131). Berlin: Springer Verlag.

Zihl, J. (1989). Cerebral disturbances of elementary visual function. In J.W. Brown (Ed.), *Neuropsychology of visual perception* (pp. 35–58). Hillsdale, NJ: Erlbaum.

Zihl, J. (1990). Treatment of patients with homonymous hemianopia. [In German]. *Zeitschrift für Neuropsychologie, 2*, 95–101.

Zihl, J. (1994). Rehabilitation of visual impairments in patients with brain damage. In A.C. Koijman, P.L. Looijesijn, J.A. Welling, & G.J. van der Wildt (Eds), *Low vision* (pp. 287–295). Amsterdam, Oxford: IOS Press.

Zihl, J. (1995a). Eye movement patterns in hemianopic dyslexia. *Brain, 118*, 891–912.

Zihl, J. (1995b). Visual scanning behavior in patients with homonymous hemianopia. *Neuropsychologia, 33*, 287–303.

Zihl, J., & Kennard, C. (1996). Disorders of higher visual function. In Th. Brandt, L.R. Caplan, J. Dichgans, H.C. Diener, & C. Kennard (Eds), *Neurological disorders: Course and treatment* (pp. 201–212). San Diego: Academic Press.

Zihl, J., & Kerkhoff, G. (1990). Foveal photopic and scotopic adaptation in patients with brain damage. *Clinical Vision Sciences, 5*, 185–195.

Zihl, J., Krischer, C., & Meissen, R. (1984). Hemianopic dyslexia and its treatment [in German]. *Nervenarzt, 55*, 317–323.

Zihl, J., & Mayer, J. (1981). Colour perimetry: Method and diagnostic value. [In German]. *Nervenarzt, 52*, 547–580.

Zihl, J., Roth, W., Kerkhoff, G., & Heywood, C.A. (1988). The influence of homonymous visual field disorders on colour sorting performance in the FM 100-hue test. *Neuropsychologia, 26,* 869–876.

Zihl, J., & von Cramon, D. (1979). The contribution of the "second" visual system to directed visual attention in man. *Brain, 102,* 835–856.

Zihl, J., & von Cramon, D. (1985). Visual field recovery from scotoma in patients with postgeniculate damage. A review of 55 cases. *Brain, 108,* 335–365.

Zihl, J., & von Cramon, D. (1986a). Recovery of visual field in patients with postgeniculate damage. In K. Poeck, H.J. Freund, & H. Gänshirt (Eds), *Neurology* (pp. 188–194). Berlin, Heidelberg: Springer.

Zihl, J., & von Cramon, D. (1986b). *Zerebrale Sehstörungen.* Stuttgart: Kohlhammer Verlag.

Zihl, J., von Cramon, D., & Mai, N. (1983). Selective disturbance of movement vision after bilateral brain damage. *Brain, 106,* 313–340.

Zihl, J., von Cramon, D., Mai, N., & Schmid, Ch. (1991). Disturbance of movement vision after bilateral posterior brain damage. Further evidence and follow up observations. *Brain, 114,* 2235–2252.

Appendix

The appendix contains a summary of and suggestions for diagnosis methods and treatment of patients with cerebral visual disorders. Before testing a patient with suspected cerebral visual disorders, a detailed neuro-ophthalmological examination is recommended to assess whether or not the peripheral visual system is also causing, for example, field defects and impaired colour vision, and to assess eye movement abnormalities (e.g. oculomotor nerve palsies).

For the assessment of practice effects, all affected visual functions and abilities (see the sections on diagnostics later) should be re-tested. Pre–post comparisons allow the differentiation between specific (only the function or ability which was subjected to treatment shows an improvement) and unspecific treatment effects.

The difficulty of tasks selected for practice should also be adapted to the initial/actual level of the patient's resources (attention, motivation).

It may very helpful for both the patient and the therapist to know the plan of treatment before the beginning of practice, and the significance of the (individual) steps with regard to the final goal. Appropriate feedback to the patient about the actual level of performance is also recommended.

HOMONYMOUS VISUAL FIELD DISORDERS

Diagnostics

Assessment should include:

Visual field mapping: Quantitative perimetry using light, colour and form targets, including accurate mapping of the degree of visual field sparing especially along the horizontal axes.

Visual scanning: Use of parallel versions of search tasks. The use of large (for example, 40° horizontal and 30° vertical) screens is recommended for the sake of ecological validity. Scanning performance can be defined in terms of scanning or searching time and number of errors (omissions, comissions). For the valid assessment of a patient's scanning behaviour, no instruction should be given how to proceed.

Reading: Reading performance can be assessed using parallel reading tests consisting of at least one page of text (for example, 20 lines, 9–10 words per line). It is recommended to use large print (for example, Univers, 12pt). Subjects are asked to read aloud, but otherwise no instruction is given on how to read. Reading performance can be defined in terms of correctly read words per minute (wpm). Self-corrections are possible and do not count as errors but will increase reading time and therefore reduce reading performance.

Reading of numbers should be assessed separately, because patients typically have greater difficulty with numbers.

Additional diagnostics

In case of suspected visual neglect standardised testing procedures for assessment should be used (e.g. Halligan et al., 1991).

Treatment

- Enlargement of saccades to the affected side(s) using a perimeter, slides, or a screen.
- Practice of visual scanning and spatial orientation using visual search tasks on slides or on a screen; gradual increase in the level of difficulty (number of items; reduction of presentation time).
- Practice of reading using tachistoscopic presentation of words, short sentences and numbers; gradual increase in the level of difficulty (increasing length of words and numbers; reduction of presentation time).

Comments

- The patient must not use head shifts before eye shifts, because it may impede the acquisition of large saccades and of oculomotor scanning strategies.
- The site and extent of posterior brain injury should be considered for the planning of treatment; patients with occipitoparietal injury or additional injury to the white matter typically need more practice.
- Patients' reports concerning the presence and absence of difficulties do not always correlate with objective testing, but are important for the assessment of patients' experience with the consequences caused by the visual field disorders and the presence or absence of awareness.

• Patients may have and report fewer or even no difficulties in familiar sur-roundings; it seems reasonable, therefore, to ask in detail for difficulties in familiar and unfamiliar surroundings.

SPATIAL CONTRAST SENSITIVITY

Diagnostics

Assessment should include:
  • Measurement of spatial contrast sensitivity.
  • Measurement of visual acuity.
  • Assessment of reading performance (see Homonymous Visual Field Disorders).

Treatment

  • Practice of spatial contrast sensitivity (e.g. three spatial frequencies)

Comments

"Blurred vision" is a common complaint that usually does not suggest any particular diagnosis. Retrochiasmatic brain injury is one cause; there is, however, a great variety of prechiasmatic causes, as for example demyelination (optic neuritis; multiple sclerosis), ischaemia, inflammations, tumours, and intoxications. Opacities of the media and refractive errors may also cause visual blurring. In cases with prechiasmatic affections, blurred vision may be restricted to one eye only; if both eyes are affected, reduction in contrast sensitivity may considerably differ between the two eyes. In patients with retrochiasmatic injury, monocular differences in contrast sensitivity are typically rather small. Patients complaining of blurred vision should always be seen by an ophthalmologist.

COLOUR VISION

Diagnostics

Assessment should include:
  • Mapping of the visual field with coloured targets.
  • Colour discrimination (FM 100-hue test).
  • Identification and recognition of objects with colours as characteristic object features.
  • Colour naming.

Treatment

  • Discrimination of colour hues.
  • Use of colours in the context of visual object identification and recognition.

VISUAL SPACE PERCEPTION

Diagnostics

Assessment should include:
  • Visual localisation in space (including saccadic and fixation accuracy as well as accuracy of visually guided grasping).
    • Discrimination of length, orientation, and size.
    • Vertical, horizontal, and straight-ahead axes.
    • Depth perception (stereopsis). ,
    • Visuoconstructive abilities (copying, drawing).
    • Reading (see Homonymous Visual Field Disorders).

Treatment

  • Practice of visual localisation in space (fixation; grasping).
  • Practice of length, size, and orientation discrimination.
  • Practice of the subjective vertical and horizontal axes.

BALINT'S SYNDROME

Diagnostics

Assessment should include:
  • Mapping of the visual field and the field of view.
  • Mapping of the field of attention and of simultaneous perception.
  • Visual orientation (in familiar and unfamiliar surroundings).
  • Visually guided grasping.
  • Visuoconstructive abilities.
  • Visual object recognition and reading.

Treatment

  • Practice of enlargement of saccadic eye movements and of visual localisation.
  • Practice of simultaneous vision.
  • "Expansion" of the field of attention by stepwise enlargement of the size of the stimulus array.
  • Practice of visual scanning and searching.
  • Practice of visual orientation.
  • Practice of the inspection of scenes and with reading.

Comments

  • Patients with severe Balint's syndrome may complain of being blind and may rely on acoustic cues to determine the position of people talking to them, and they may use tactile cues to find their way even in their familiar surroundings. It should therefore always be taken into account which modality actually "offers" the patient more safety and independence.

• After the improvement in using visual information, patients quite often have to be gently "forced" to use their regained visual abilities for visual orientation at least in familiar surroundings.

• Patients with severely impaired or lost topographical memory may not be able to do so because they can no longer reliably store spatial and topographical information. In these cases, improvement of oculomotor scanning and widening of the field of attention may not be sufficient.

VISUAL RECOGNITION

Diagnostics

Assessment should include:

• "Elementary" visual functions and abilities which are prerequisites for visual identification and recognition (visual fields, visual acuity, and contrast sensitivity, colour vision, visual scanning, fixation accuracy).
• Visual recognition of objects, faces, letters, and numbers.
• Reading and writing.

Treatment

• If required, improvement of "elementary" visual functions and abilities which are prerequisites of visual identification and recognition.
• Practice of category-specific visual recognition, including.
    (1) processing of object attributes.
    (2) selection of object properties.
    (3) supervision of visual identification/recognition processes.
    (4) association of visual stimuli with proper descriptions (names, labels).
• In patients with alexia: practice of reading.

Comments

It is important to consider difficulties with visual naming which could interfere with the report of visual identification and recognition.

CENTRAL SCOTOMA

Diagnostics

Assessment should include:
• Visual field mapping.
• Contrast sensitivity and visual acuity.
• Spatial localisation (fixation accuracy; grasping).
• Visual recognition and reading.

Treatment

- Practice of localisation accuracy (saccadic accuracy and fixation accuracy).
- Practice of spatial resolution and form discrimination.
- Practice of visual recognition.
- Practice of reading.

Comments

- Depending on the size of the central scotoma and the associated visual deficits, practice should be started either with a task requiring the localisation of single stimuli or with form discrimination (in cases with fairly preserved fixation accuracy).
- It seems important for patients to use their impaired vision even for only "crude" visual orientation and localisation as soon as possible in familiar surroundings, especially when no further spatial (topographical agnosia) or cognitive (memory) disorders are present.

Author Index

181

Subject Index